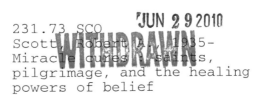

Miracle Cures

The publisher gratefully acknowledges the generous support of the Ahmanson Foundation Humanities Endowment Fund of the University of California Press Foundation.

The publisher also gratefully acknowledges the generous support of William and Sheila Nolan as members of the Literati Circle of the University of California Press Foundation.

Miracle Cures

*Saints, Pilgrimage, and
the Healing Powers of Belief*

Robert A. Scott

UNIVERSITY OF CALIFORNIA PRESS

Berkeley   Los Angeles   London

University of California Press, one of the most distinguished
university presses in the United States, enriches lives around
the world by advancing scholarship in the humanities, social
sciences, and natural sciences. Its activities are supported by
the UC Press Foundation and by philanthropic contributions from individuals and institutions. For more information, visit www.ucpress.edu.

University of California Press
Berkeley and Los Angeles, California

University of California Press, Ltd.
London, England

Library of Congress Cataloging-in-Publication Data

Scott, Robert A., 1935–.
    Miracle cures : saints, pilgrimage, and the healing powers
of belief / Robert A. Scott.
        p.   cm.
    Includes bibliographical references and index.
    ISBN 978-0-520-26275-1 (cloth : alk. paper)
    1. Spiritual healing.   2. Healing—Religious aspects—
Christianity.   3. Miracles.   I. Title.
BT732.5.S34   2010
    231.7'3—dc22

                                              2009037269

Manufactured in the United States of America

19 18 17 16 15 14 13 12 11 10
10 9 8 7 6 5 4 3 2 1

This book is printed on Cascades Enviro 100, a 100% post
consumer waste, recycled, de-inked fiber. FSC recycled
certified and processed chlorine free. It is acid free, Ecologo
certified, and manufactured by BioGas energy.

To Julia,
and for Jane, Winfield, Tom, and Nonie

CONTENTS

PART TWO / SAINTS AND HEALING

ILLUSTRATIONS

FIGURES

MAP

ACKNOWLEDGMENTS

It is a pleasure to acknowledge the people and the institutions that provided me with invaluable assistance and support as I was researching and writing this book. I begin with New College, Oxford, where I was privileged to spend the Hilary term of 2005 as a visiting fellow. I am deeply grateful to Alan Ryan, the warden of New College, and Miles Hewstone, fellow of the college, for accommodating me and my wife, Julia, during the term, and to the Bodleian Library, where I spent productive hours immersed in its outstanding medieval collections. Oxford University and its magnificent library provide ideal environments for conducting scholarly research and writing, and I consider myself truly privileged to have spent a term in residence there. I also thank Ruth Harris, another fellow of the college, for her assistance in guiding me through materials about Lourdes.

I have also benefited from access to other libraries whose collections have been indispensable to my research. They include the British Library in London, the Stanford University Library, and the library at Salisbury Cathedral. I especially thank the cathedral's librarian, Suzanne Eward, for generously making materials concerning Saint Osmund available for my inspection.

The Center for Advanced Study in the Behavioral Sciences at Stanford University helped me immensely in developing and advancing my ideas. Early on in my project I benefited greatly from participation in a special project on art, mind, and the brain that was sponsored by the center during the 2001–2 academic year. My thinking was also enriched by conversations with a number of former fellows of the center, including Dan Carpenter, Robert Ader, Bill Christian, Gabor Klaniczay, and Ann Taves. I especially thank Chandra Mukerji and other members of the object and agency discussion group that convened during the 2008–9 fellowship year. Beyond this, the center, where I served as associate director from 1983 to 2001, provided an ideal setting for interdisciplinary study.

The medievalist John Hatcher of Cambridge University provided me with helpful descriptions of life during the Middle Ages. Margo Horn supplied much-appreciated help with materials about women in medieval society. Nancy Adler offered help and advice on large segments of part 2 of this book, as did her colleague Margaret Kemeny, whose work on shame and health is central to sections of chapter 6. I also benefited from an extended conversation with the dermatologist Owen Stier about placebo responses to common skin conditions. Jeremy Medina helped me to gain access to the Spanish monastery at Toribio to examine its famous relic, a portion of the true cross. In addition, Jeremy and his wife Jackie led a tour of northern Spain that Julia and I were privileged to join, which included visits to many of its great cathedral shrines. Erica Goode and Alana Connor read earlier drafts of my manuscript and offered deft editorial advice. I am especially grateful to Don Lamm for his guidance throughout, especially during the publication process, and to Neil Smelser, who I later learned had served as a reader of this manuscript for the University of California Press. A second reader, this one anonymous, provided important suggestions that have helped bring balance to my argument.

John Mustain, head of the Special Collections Division of the Stanford University Library, assisted me in locating illustrations for the book, as did Evelyn McMillan. Alan Howard, Jan Renzel, and Kathleen Much offered advice on a title for the book.

As is the custom in acknowledgments, I should add that I bear sole responsibility for content of the book and for any errors of interpretation it may contain. (Truth to tell, I would much prefer to accept credit for all praise and assign all blame to others, but, alas, my editor advises that this would be bad form.)

Which brings me to my editor. Reed Malcolm, senior acquisitions editor at the University of California Press, has been encouraging and supportive of this project from the beginning, offering sage advice at every step of the way and applying his editorial and managerial skills to help bring the project to publication. Thanks also to Erika Büky, who did a masterful job of copyediting.

This book was conceived and written in the context of my participation with the Sarum Seminar, an ongoing gathering of individuals from all walks of life in the San Francisco Bay Area who have a common interest in medieval matters. We have been meeting on a regular basis for nearly fifteen years to hear talks, plan trips together, and engage in research. The nearly sixty active members of the seminar have been a source of advice, encouragement, and inspiration throughout, and I acknowledge and thank them for their enthusiastic interest and support.

Finally, this book could not have been written or ever seen the light of day without the help of my wife, Julia Fremon. She has performed with consummate skill as editor, critic, researcher, and protector of my time, my vision of the ideal soulmate and life companion, to whom I gratefully dedicate this work.

PROLOGUE

On December 14, 1421, in the English city of Salisbury, a fourteen-year-old girl named Agnes suffered a grievous injury when a hot spit pierced her torso. Bystanders managed to extract the spit, but her condition remained grave. She was all but given up for dead when her parents, along with several neighbors, prayed to Osmund, the eleventh-century bishop of Sarum (modern-day Salisbury), whose tomb was in Salisbury Cathedral. At the time, Osmund was still a saint-in-waiting; though he had been proposed for canonization in 1228, he was not officially canonized until 1457. In their prayers, the supplicants vowed to Osmund that if Agnes's life was spared, they would visit his tomb, honor him in prayer, and leave gifts in thanks for his miraculous intercession with God on the child's behalf. Shortly thereafter, Agnes began to show renewed signs of life. Two days after regaining consciousness, she rose from her bed and walked around her house, and ten days after that she was described as completely recovered.[1] The event was duly noted in documents submitted by the dean and chapter of Salisbury Cathedral to the Roman Curia (the Vatican's judicial court) in support of Osmund's canonization.

This was one of fifty-two miracles attributed to Osmund. According to a petition to the curia by a commission representing Salisbury Cathedral in 1423, two years after Agnes's miraculous recovery, Osmund had a direct hand in curing paralysis, restoring sanity to a madman, restoring the sight of a blind person, relieving pain caused by injuries, and curing illnesses of various kinds.[2]

At roughly the same time but in a different part of Europe, another miracle occurred, involving one Guibert of Burgundy. Several years earlier, Guibert had lost the use of his legs. He set off by cart for Santiago de Compostela, at the far northeastern corner of Spain—a thousand kilometers from his home—to visit the famous shrine of Christ's apostle Saint James. Guibert was housed in a hospital near the basilica, where priests counseled him to pray to the saint. He kept a vigil in the church for two nights, and on the third he claimed that a figure appeared to him, took his hand, and raised him up. When the pilgrim asked the figure to identify himself, he replied, "I am James, the apostle of God." Guibert was immediately restored to health. He kept a vigil for thirteen more days in the church and then began to travel about the countryside telling people what had happened to him.[3]

Reports about saints performing similar miracles during the medieval period are legion. They are said to have cured afflictions of every kind—blindness, deafness, dumbness, paralysis, chronic pain, fever, stomach ailments, leprosy—and even to have raised the dead. Indeed, canonization for a holy figure was not even considered by the Church unless the candidate was known to have performed miraculous cures.

One of medieval England's most important saints, Thomas Becket, the famously martyred archbishop of Canterbury, was slain in his own cathedral on December 29, 1170. John of Salisbury (1115 or 1120–80), who had served as Becket's personal secretary and later became bishop of Chartres Cathedral in France, wrote about the experiences of pilgrims who visited Becket's shrine: "For in the place of his passion, and in the place where he lay before the great altar previous to burial, and in the place where he was at last buried, paralytics are cured, the blind see, the deaf hear, the dumb speak, the lame walk, lepers are cured. . . . And the dead are raised . . . the deformed [are] well formed; he causes gout and fever to be cured; drop-sied and leprous folk he restores . . . and [causes] the mad to return to their senses."[4] Few modern-day physicians can boast of such accomplishments.

Belief in the possibility of miraculous cures through the agency of a saint is not restricted to the medieval period. Though less widely accepted today than it once was, the idea that saints can perform mir-acles enjoyed considerable currency long after the Enlightenment and remains very much alive today. Most readers have heard about Lourdes in the French Pyrenees, where the Virgin Mary appeared to the peas-ant girl Bernadette Soubirous in 1857; it now attracts several million pilgrims and other visitors each year. According to one source, in 2001 more than six million people visited Lourdes, including many who were sick and seeking the intercession of the Virgin to effect a cure.[5]

Among the sixty-six miracles at Lourdes recognized by the Catholic Church is one that involved a woman named Virginie Gordet in 1892. She suffered from an undiagnosed muscular disorder that hampered her ability to walk. The official account of her miracle reads as follows:

On contact with the water [from the famous grotto], the sick woman said: "Lord, may your will be done." It seemed to her that her limbs were relaxing, that their strength was returning. But she dared not yet believe and went on repeating: "Saint Mary, pray for me! Blessed Virgin, cure me!" The women who assisted her were moved to the depths of their souls! At their suggestion, and without any indication of difficulty or suffering, Mme. Gordet took a few steps in the piscine, then, alone, submerged herself a second time. "But you are cured!" exclaimed the ladies. "Ah! Help me, Mesdames, to thank the Blessed Virgin!" Then the woman, Virginie Gordet, reportedly walked up the three steps of the pool alone, holding her crutches, and, while she threw herself at the feet of the statue of the Virgin with her *visage transfiguré*, onlookers in the bathhouse began to say the *Magnificat*.[6]

Those of us whose notions about the causes and cures of sickness are rooted in medical science may have difficulty knowing what to make of such reports. Often they are dismissed as exaggerations, even pure fictions, born of wishful or misguided thinking on the part of uneducated, superstitious people desperate for relief from suffering.[7] I do not share this view.

Some deeply religious people understand illness and cure as evidence of direct divine intervention in human affairs. Others, equally devout, find it difficult to accept such claims uncritically. I leave it to them to debate this aspect of miracle cures. I propose an additional explanation for what happens when people of faith and belief appeal to saints for relief from bodily suffering. It is based on a body of theory and research that has been largely overlooked by those who study miracle cures: the work of social, behavioral, and medical scientists showing that culture, beliefs, cognitions, emotions, social relationships, and physical environment play a central role in the onset, course, and outcome of illness. I do not dismiss, negate, or supplant the views of religious believers but instead extend the modern understanding of what transpires in the body and mind when the faithful report that they gain relief from their suffering by appealing to saints.

My only real quarrel is with those who dismiss all such claims of cure as hogwash. Even while making allowances for exaggeration, wishful thinking, and shameless propaganda, I nevertheless conclude that if a sufferer claims to have obtained relief by appealing to a saint, that person's account has validity. In the eyes of some medical scientists, these cures may be illusory, in the sense that they are not always permanent, but there are nonetheless solid scientific grounds for the claims of supplicants that their practices can provide relief from suffering. In other words, I argue that the faithful feel confident in appealing to saints for cures because for certain conditions, and under certain circumstances, such appeals actually work.

I draw on insights by social and behavioral scientists who have studied the cultural, cognitive, and situational bases for health and illness. Belief in the power of saints to cure, participation in the practices associated with pilgrimage, and engagement in acts of veneration of saints at shrines where their relics are housed combine to instill in many pilgrims a distinct experience of feeling better. For some illnesses, such acts may give rise to physiological processes that can lead to lasting recovery.

BACKGROUND

In 2003 I published a book about the medieval Gothic cathedrals of Europe.[8] In it I address questions that often cross the minds of visitors: How did the people of medieval Europe manage to build such audacious structures? Why did they do so? What were the buildings for? Behind these and similar questions lies a puzzle. The economy of Europe during the Middle Ages was based largely on subsistence farming.[9] How could resource-deprived, underdeveloped, technologically primitive communities, barely surviving from one harvest to the next, manage to create magnificent works of architecture like the cathedrals of Chartres, Notre Dame, and Canterbury? Why would anyone think such undertakings a prudent use of scarce liquid capital? To what worthwhile communal purposes was a cathedral put?

Answering these questions required me to investigate—among other things—where the cathedral builders found funds to underwrite the costs of construction and maintenance. Cathedral-building projects were colossal sinkholes for liquid capital at a time when the supply was meager and the demands on it varied and urgent. How was the money to build a Chartres or a Canterbury Cathedral raised?

The bishops who built Europe's medieval cathedrals amassed the funds to build and maintain them in just about any way they could. I won't review their methods here, except to mention one that especially intrigued me. For at least some cathedrals—though not for all—one substantial source of revenue was gifts left by pilgrims at the shrines of saints at the cathedral site.[10] Those seeking cures showed their admiration for the saints to whom they appealed for relief by making gifts, and the most common gift was coins. (In medieval England the expected amount was one penny.) Such gifts could generate a small but steady revenue stream to help underwrite the enormous costs of building and maintaining a cathedral.[11]

Pilgrimages to the shrines of great saints contributed to the accumulation of capital in other ways as well. Substantial revenues, many of which the bishops were able to tax, were generated by activities such as the great fairs and markets held on or around saints' feast days. These revenues were not nearly enough to cover the costs of building or renovating a great cathedral, but they certainly helped.

More than any other in England, Canterbury Cathedral's shrine to Thomas Becket exemplified the financial benefit to a cathedral or church of securing the relics of a saint, gaining renown as a place where miracles occurred, and thereby becoming a popular pilgrimage destination. The medievalist Ben Nilson, who has conducted a comprehensive study of cathedral-affiliated pilgrimage shrines in medieval England, reports that on certain special occasions, crowds of more than one hundred thousand people reportedly gathered at the cathedral to honor Becket.[12] A crowd of this size is not all that unusual today (Wembley Stadium, the site of major soccer matches in London, can seat ninety thousand), but imagine for a moment what such a gathering would have represented in thirteenth-century England. Suppose, for the sake of illustration, that 75 percent of all of the visitors to Canterbury came from England and Wales, which evidence suggests is a reasonable guess. The total combined population of England and Wales at that time probably did not exceed five or six million people; thus roughly 1 out of every 66 to 80 citizens came to Canterbury on important occasions.[13]

Surviving account books indicate that such crowds helped generate impressive sums of money, which were placed at the disposal of the monastic order at Canterbury Cathedral. During the first half of the thirteenth century, the annual yield from gifts left by pilgrims at Becket's shrine is estimated to have been about one thousand pounds, a fortune at the time. Account books for the year 1220 show that gifts from pilgrims made up almost two-thirds of the total income of the monastery, and records for 1275 show that the shrine was the hub of Canterbury Cathedral's fiscal activities. Its keepers routinely extended grants to other units of the cathedral, especially its works department.[14]

Among the things that swelled this source of revenue were the widely publicized claims made by Canterbury monks and others about miracles at Becket's shrine. The same was true at other saints' shrines. Nearly all of Europe's great cathedrals aspired to attract sick people who came to pray for a miraculous cure. It was this potential of saints as fundraisers for cathedral and other ecclesiastical building projects that first piqued my curiosity about miracle cures. In particular, why did people in this period of history feel so certain that visits to saints' shrines and worship of their relics might cure illness? What experiences buttressed their belief in these claims to the point where people, many of them poor peasants, were prepared to undertake arduous journeys and part with their hard-earned money? And why does this belief persist today?

The world of contemporary Christianity is populated with famous healing shrines: Lourdes, Compostela, Fátima in Portugal, La Salette in the French Alps, Medjugorje in Bosnia, Chimayo in New Mexico (sometimes referred to as "the Lourdes of America"), Sainte Anne de Beaupré in Canada, the shrine to Saint Anne d'Auray in Brittany, the shrine to Our Lady of Guadalupe north of Mexico City—the list goes on and on. Though no comprehensive census tells us exactly how many people visit these places each year, they number in the many millions. To be sure, only a fraction of today's visitors are actually ailing and in search of cures. Many more visit these sites as companions to the ill, on spiritual quests, or out of a sense of obligation to their faith. But regardless of their reasons for going, pilgrimages to the shrines of important saints are a major industry today, and the vast stream of *malades* who journey to Lourdes each year powerfully attests to the continued vibrancy of belief in the healing power of holy figures.

MIRACLE CURES AND MODERN SCIENCE

Proponents of modern scientific medicine, of whom I am one, are mystified by some of the claims that are made about acts of miraculous healing at the shrines of saints. Western understanding about the causes of disease is, of course, deeply rooted in biology. For this reason, the idea of miracle cures meets with widespread skepticism. We wonder how the Virgin Mary and the Christian saints, and the shrines dedicated to them, could possibly have anything to do with treating sickness. While we admit that devotional practices offer comfort to those who suffer, we see nothing in such practices that seems even remotely relevant to effecting a cure—unless the condition is hysterical or psychosomatic in nature. The essence of science-based medicine is the use of tests and technologies—the X-ray, the MRI, the CAT scan, the EEG, the EKG, the biopsy, the stress test, chemical blood and urine tests—to identify and diagnose symptoms, and then the use of drugs, surgery, and other physiology-based therapies to treat their underlying causes. Healing shrines offer only the power of the saints and their relics. What effect can strands of hair, pieces of bone, finger- and toenail clippings, teeth, and shreds of a saint's clothing possibly have on an ailing body? The two worlds could hardly be more different, and we should not be surprised to find that proponents of scientific medicine often view the world of healing shrines with deep skepticism.

One purpose of this book is to try to bring these two worlds closer together. I hope to shed light on why the impulse best expressed in the oft-quoted phrase from Chaucer's *Canterbury Tales*—"The holy blessed martyr St. Thomas à Becket, who helped them when they were sick"—strikes so many of the faithful as plausible.[15]

Understanding Miracle Cures

It is easy to reject the miracle cure as nonsense, to dismiss it as a false conclusion born of desperation and based on incorrect inferences rooted in ignorance, superstition, hearsay, speculation, and misinformation. While in certain instances this view is probably warranted, I nevertheless wondered how the cult of saints as an institution, with its attendant practices, could have survived and flourished throughout the Middle Ages, and until today, if it were based on ignorance alone. It seemed to me that there had to be more to the story than just ignorance and stupidity.

I began reading about the medieval cult of saints, in particular examining reports of miracle cures said to have taken place at healing shrines in medieval England and elsewhere in Europe. I sought not only a fuller understanding of all aspects of the medieval cult of saints but also a better feel for what people meant when they spoke of miracle cures, and in particular to learn about the sorts of physical conditions for which pilgrims had claimed benefits. At the same time, I investigated what is known about patterns of morbidity (i.e., rates of death from various causes) in medieval European communities. I read accounts of what pilgrimage entailed and what awaited pilgrims at the shrines. Did things happen en route and at the pilgrims' destinations, I wondered, that might help explain why they believed their health was improving? And I looked for materials that might shed light on what prompted sick people to become pilgrims in the first place, what beliefs led them to turn to saints for help, and what demeanors and behaviors were expected of them in connection with pilgrimage and appealing for a cure.

As I sifted through this information, I began to sense the potential relevance of work done by biomedical, social, and behavioral scientists on factors implicated in illness. I was generally familiar with this domain of research, having previously taught courses on the subject to Princeton and Stanford undergraduates, and over the years I have tried to keep up with developments in these fields. It seemed to me that by merging insights gained from this research with what I was learning about pilgrimage and worship of saints, I could add to our understanding of why people felt they had been cured, offering an explanation for their experiences that was more plausible and interesting than accounts attributing their experiences to ignorance and superstition alone.

I am scarcely the first to point out why a pilgrimage might contribute to a sick person's sense of well-being. Changes in diet, climate, and daily routine associated with traveling to pilgrimage shrines might all have beneficial effects, together with the powerful experience of being with others with a common purpose.[16] But recent research on health and illness can also add to our understanding of what may have been taking place. Studies have demonstrated the positive effects of thought processes (i.e., cognitions) on the immune system; the ways cognitive framing and the focus of attention can shape people's awareness and experience of how they feel, particularly their experience of pain; the role of belief in people's responses to treatment regimens (commonly called the placebo effect); the healing power of emotional expression; the beneficial effects that personal initiative can have on the immune system; and the role that hope born of belief can play in coping with and diminishing pain, reducing inflammation, allaying anxiety, and ameliorating depression.

My project entails an attempt to anneal traditions of scholarship that until now have developed largely independently of one another. One tradition is the work by historians, scholars of religion, theologians, spiritualists and others on medieval and modern-day healing shrines. The other is contemporary biomedical, social, and behavioral-science research that investigates how cultural, social, and personal factors influence illness and recovery. In each of these traditions, the questions that are asked, the kinds of data that are sought and are available for analysis, the methods employed in gathering them, the ways they are interpreted—and, for that matter, what counts as relevant evidence—are often alien, sometimes even repugnant, to members of the other camp. Annealing these two traditions requires proponents on each side to adopt an open and tolerant frame of mind. Humanists need to suspend whatever doubts they may harbor about positivist science in general and social science in particular. For their part, biomedical and other scientists need to understand that despite the nearly complete absence of independently verifiable, quantitative empirical data about the physical ailments afflicting visitors to medieval healing shrines, it is nevertheless possible to draw meaningful inferences about peoples' illnesses and recoveries from the evidence that has survived. Those who insist that the only valid statements that can be made about human illness are those based on modern clinical-study methods will be disappointed by what follows. By stating these differences at the outset, I hope to persuade proponents of both views to lay their weapons aside, as it were, and prepare to listen to one another with open and understanding minds.

DISCLAIMERS

The approach I adopt does not purport to explain all miraculous events. Some of the cures I have read about frankly mystify me. If they are accurate accounts of what actually transpired, then I can think of no plausible explanation based in medical science. But for a majority of the events about which I have read, I believe many of the factors identified by social and behavioral science research can help to explain why people become ill and subsequently recover. I attempt to apply the findings of this research to explain what happens when people who are ill approach saints for cures, and why doing so may help them feel better and in some cases actually recover.

Readers might suspect me of dismissing all faith-based explanations for miracle cures in favor of those based on the findings of scientific medical research. They are wrong. Though I do not consider myself a religious person, I respect the views of those who believe that spirituality, the spiritual quest, faith, devotion to God, and religious experience play an important role in what transpires when people appeal to saints for relief. These matters have long been a source of interest, fascination, amazement, and awe to theologians, scientists, and laypeople. Indeed, one need only search the Internet, using phrases such as "healing and prayer," "religion and healing," or "healing and devotion," to find millions upon millions of entries; or to search the lists of books by such well-known authors as Phil Cousineau, Robert Torrance, Joseph Campbell, Bill Moyers, Lauren Artress, Bruce Chatwin, and others to appreciate the depth and breadth of the conviction that spirituality and healing are tightly linked.[17]

What I have to say on the topic is not meant to supersede the views of writers such as these on the matter or to dispute their accounts. It is meant, instead, to complement them by bringing to bear on the topic of healing bodies of scientific theory and research that I believe can help us to understand what transpires when people pray to the saints for healing.

There are at least two different senses in which I regard my treatment of the subject as complementary to theirs. One is to shed light on how acts of miraculous healing actually happen. Surely even the most ardent believer would accept that when a cure for an illness occurs in connection with venerating a saint, both the mind and the body are involved. I identify bodies of theory and research that provide important clues for understanding what happens inside the minds and under the skins of people who report being healed through the agency of saints.

Second, as I have explained elsewhere and reiterate later in this book,[18] it has long been the practice in the Catholic Church to carefully scrutinize claims of miracle cures, turning to medical science to rule out the possibility of naturalistic explanations before entertaining the idea that a healing event might be the result of divine intervention. Thus, at Lourdes today, the Vatican convenes panels of medical experts who study each case in detail in an effort to either identify or rule out natural causes for cures. The expertise to which Church authorities turn is typically drawn from established medical specialties. This is as it should be; but the specialties represented are not well-known for incorporating social and behavioral science research into their understanding of illness. I believe my findings might inform deliberations by medical experts who are assigned the task of identifying and ruling out false positives. Incorporating them would increase the credibility of those deliberations that find no apparent naturalistic cause for the episodes of illness.

Another disclaimer concerns pilgrimage. Although I focus here on the practice of pilgrimage in the Christian faith, I recognize that pilgrimage is common to many other great religions.[19] In Islam, for example, the pilgrimage to Mecca, a reenactment of the pilgrimage made by Muhammad three months before his death, is considered the supreme expression of faith.[20] Known as the hajj, it draws travelers of every description; to quote from Michael Wolfe's account, they include "poets, bureaucrats, spies, ne'er-do-wells, queens, slaves, the fabulously wealthy, old and young, lawyers, judges, confidence men, scholars, novelists, existentialists, and devout believers . . . Persians, Moroccans, Afghans, Meccans, Spaniards, Australians, Hindi Indians, Austrians, Italians, Swiss, Americans and British."[21] For fourteen centuries Mecca has been a spiritual destination for millions of men and women the world over; today it attracts more than two million pilgrims each year. Wolfe explains that the point of the hajj has remained much the same since its inception: "To detach a representative number of people from their homes and, by bringing them to Islam's birthplace, to emphasize the unity of all human beings before their creator."[22] All Muslims are required to go on hajj once during their lives.

Pilgrimage is a central part of religious practice among Hindus as well.[23] One of the terms often used to describe Hindu pilgrimages is *tirthas*, a Sanskrit word connoting a ford and thus the idea of metaphorically crossing between the human and the divine. For Hindus, the most monumental pilgrimage is Kumbh Mela, which occurs four times every twelve years and rotates among four locations: Prayag (Allahabad), Haridwar, Ujjain, and Nashit. The Great (Purna or Maha) Kumbh Mela takes place at Allahabad every twelve years. According to one source, the 2001 Kumbh Mela at Allahabad attracted some eight million pilgrims, and the Great Kumbh Mela has been known to attract as many as seventy million, making it the largest gathering for any purpose anywhere in the world.[24] The medieval pilgrimages to Canterbury pale in comparison to the Great Kumbh Mela. Worldwide there are an estimated 837 million adherents of Hinduism, so on average about 1 of every 12 Hindus participates.

Buddhists, too, go on pilgrimage. The Buddha spoke of four places to which followers should make a pilgrimage: Lumbini, where he was born; Bodh Gaya, where he attained enlightenment; Sarnath, where he preached his first sermon; and Kusinara, where he died.[25] These, along with four other destinations, constitute the so-called Eight Great Places of pilgrimage in India and Nepal, all of them attracting tens of thousands of pilgrims at a time. There are less famous but equally well-attended Buddhist pilgrimage shrines in Afghanistan, Cambodia, China, Indonesia, Japan, Laos, Myanmar, South Korea, Thailand, and Tibet.

The practices of pilgrimage in the Islamic, Buddhist, Hindu, and Christian faiths may have different destinations and objectives, but are all expressions of a deep spiritual quest. These practices also often express a shared thirst for healing: the connection of pilgrimage and miracles is not unique to Christianity. However, their specific roles in other religions are beyond the scope of this book.

My own inquiry, then, is not about pilgrimages the world over, nor does it purport to deal with all aspects of religious experience or all the pilgrimages associated with Christianity.[26] I seek to understand one specific aspect of the overall experience: the miracle cures that take place in connection with appeals made by the faithful to the saints. I do not wish to suggest that miracle cures are unrelated to larger questions about spiritual quests, or that one can isolate events of healing and analyze them outside a spiritual context. What I am trying to understand is how the beliefs and rituals surrounding pilgrimage may contribute to a genuine sense of improved well-being.

PLAN OF THE BOOK

My inquiry is organized into two parts. The first is devoted to explaining the critical importance of the saints in Western European Christianity and how saints' potential to heal has been realized. I address four key questions: What were the forces within these societies that gave rise to such a powerful reliance on saints for protection and relief? This is the topic of chapter 1. I then ask what qualities and attributes are ascribed to saints that make it possible for them to play the role assigned to them, and when and how people experienced the saints' presence. Finally, I ask what people thought they had to do to access and activate the saints' powers to protect and heal. These topics are taken up in chapters 2, 3, and 4, respectively.

Part 2 explores the relevance of these findings for the health of those who participated in the cult of saints. In chapter 5, I examine what is known about the kinds of illness in medieval Europe for which miracle cures were claimed. In the subsequent three chapters I examine biomedical, social, and behavioral science research on illness to demonstrate the likely implications for recovery of such factors as beliefs about the agency of saints as facilitators of miracles, participation in the practices of veneration, and activities associated with visiting saints' shrines. Specifically, chapter 6 discusses the relationship of stress, the emotions, and shame to illness, and the role that social support plays in the response to medical treatment. Chapter 7 examines research on placebos and analgesia to explore the effects of beliefs on responses to treatment, in particular the relevance of belief to the relief of pain and discomfort. Chapter 8 examines research on factors that determine our awareness of and responses to physical symptoms, and the benefits to the immune system of talking about personal traumas as well as acting affirmatively in the face of major challenges in our lives.

A final section, the coda, presents a hypothetical scenario showing how a medieval believer might have benefited from pilgrimage and appeals to a saint. It also explores how my discussion of miracle cures is linked to past efforts to understand the so-called mind-body problem and investigates the influence of electronic media on the age-old practice of venerating saints in hopes of being cured.

PART ONE

Appealing to Saints for Miracles

CHAPTER ONE

Life in the Middle Ages

The German sociologist Max Weber once wrote: "The most elementary forms of behavior motivated by religious . . . factors are oriented to this world."[1] He identifies one of religion's most important functions as offering the hope of protection and relief from suffering and distress. The historian Michael Goodich identifies one of the key implications of Weber's insight when he writes: "The supernatural tends to intercede when human mechanisms, such as the state, prove unreliable or flawed, and the brutalization of human relations demands outside intervention to achieve equity."[2] These views imply that the appetite for divine protection and miracles among large segments of the populace is whetted when conditions of daily living are especially harsh and when society's institutions fail to protect people from the resulting dangers.[3] Such insights offer a useful framework for discussing the role of religion and saints among Western European Christians during the medieval and early modern periods.[4]

Modern Westerners sometimes describe medieval life as "nasty, brutish and short," a phrase borrowed from the seventeenth-century philosopher Thomas Hobbes to describe life as it would be in a state of nature, without law, order, or government.[5] This pithy phrase is accurate in many respects, but it obscures an important point. When we look back on medieval times from the vantage point of the twenty-first century, we tend to focus on the things that we have that were lacking then: amenities, technologies, conveniences, public services, and civic institutions that most of us take completely for granted and consider essential to our existence. From this perspective, it is inevitable that medieval life will appear bleak, harsh and dreary. But in the absence of any notion held by medieval people about what twenty-first century life might be like, things may not have seemed so bad to them. (Historians writing in the year 3010 might be similarly perplexed at how we could possibly have enjoyed life in the early twenty-first century, which might strike them as quaint and deprived.)

The Hobbesian depiction of medieval life also discounts features of communal and religious life that served as buffers against adversity, like the comfort and reassurance afforded by religion, the certain belief that divine beings could provide protection, the powerful experience of community (a major benefit of communal existence), and the sense of mutual support and obligation toward other people. These are things that gave meaning to medieval life and helped cushion people against the burden of uncertainty and the precariousness of day-to-day existence. If life was at times frightening and dangerous, it also offered sources of comfort and solace.

The first section of this chapter explains the conditions during the medieval period that made life so difficult.[6] The second describes how community and religion together offered buffers against these harsh conditions. These aspects of medieval life help us understand the roles saints played as protectors and healers of the sick.

CHALLENGES OF MEDIEVAL LIFE
Rural Living

Economic historians estimate that until about the late fifteenth century, more than 90 percent of the population lived by the planting, tending, and harvesting of crops. Subsistence farming entailed constant devotion to producing the food necessary for survival, and to meeting farmers' obligations to landowners.[7]

The amount of land available to peasant families for cultivation varied markedly. In the early fourteenth century, as the population grew, agricultural lands were repeatedly subdivided (a process known as morseling), but after the Black Death the process was reversed, and lands were once again consolidated into larger allotments.[8] The most fortunate, known as yardlanders or virgaters, farmed ten to forty acres of land, with average allotments being about twenty acres. A typical household consisted of five people: husband, wife, and three children ages 5–12.[9] Yardlanders grew grains, legumes, and perhaps a few vegetables. On average, a third of the land was planted with wheat, half with barley, and the remainder with oats, peas, and other crops.[10] The family's basic food needs for a year, mainly bread and pottage (a starchy stew made of vegetables, mainly peas and beans, and sometimes bits of meat or fish) could be met with 53 bushels of wheat, barley, and oats, plus another 24 bushels of barley for brewing ale.[11] A good wheat harvest might yield 8 to 12.5 bushels of wheat per acre (the comparable figure today is 47 bushels). However, 2.3 bushels of that yield had to be set aside for planting next year's crop. Thus, the effective wheat yield per acre in a good year was in the range of 5.7 to 10.2 bushels. The average yardlander planted a little over six acres of what, with a total yield of 38 to 68 bushels.[12]

Bread was the main food staple, constituting an estimated 82 percent of daily caloric intake. It is estimated that a single bushel of wheat, mixed with other grains, provides enough flour for 73 one-pound loaves of bread.[13] Thirty-eight bushels of wheat per harvest would produce enough wheat to make about 2,774 one-pound loaves of bread; a higher yield might produce enough for nearly five thousand loaves.[14]

A family of five needed approximately 11,000 calories per day. The adult male in the family, doing the hard work of farming, needed an estimated 2,900 calories. His wife would need at least 2,150 calories, and each of the children would need at least 2,000 calories per day. A one-pound loaf of bread contained about 1,000 calories, so a typical family needed a minimum of nine loaves of bread per day (i.e., 82 percent of 11,000, or 9,020). In a good year, the land would provide enough grain for this quantity of bread and perhaps even leave a small surplus to sell. But a poor harvest would leave the family going hungry if other sources of food could not be found.[15]

This was life for the typical yardlander. But nearly half of all holdings in the Midlands and south of England through the High Middle Ages were considerably smaller, consisting of perhaps five to ten acres of land.[16] Farmers on these lands, known as half-yardlanders, could not hope to produce sufficient food to live on. Even in good years, a ten-acre allotment, one-third of which was planted in wheat, would yield enough grain for only eight loaves of bread per day, leaving the household 12 percent short of its estimated daily calorie requirement. Thus many poor people were chronically undernourished.[17]

Daily existence, then, was highly uncertain, often unnervingly so. The production and consumption of food overwhelmed all other matters. The economic historian Carlo Cipolla explains: "The poorer the country, the greater the proportion of available income its inhabitants have to spend on food. . . . [T]he lower the income, the higher will be the percentage spent on 'poor' items such as bread and other starchy foods."[18] He estimates that between 60 and 80 percent of total income was spent on food.

The figures for crop yields that I have cited apply to harvests during good years. But even slight seasonal variations—a single storm, an unexpected dry spell, a late frost after spring planting, or an early frost at harvest—could plunge an entire community into an economic tailspin. Such events were unsettlingly common. Discussing the *Chronica Majora*, by Matthew Paris, which covers the years 1236–59, the historian Malcolm Barber comments: "No year passes . . . without some comment on rain and floods, on drought, on wind and storms, on frost, hail and snow, on the state of the air and atmospheric disturbances, on the tides, on earthquakes . . . [and] . . . on disease among humans and animals."[19] Another source, describing the years 1086–1348, speaks of the "precariousness of life, deriving . . . from man's dependence on the weather and his vulnerabilities to disease."[20]

Though few people seem to have actually starved to death, malnutrition was endemic. Chronic malnutrition, of course, heightened susceptibility to disease. Thus fevers, flu, and even the common cold were widespread and often life-threatening. Even worse, to stay alive during periods of extreme food shortage, especially in winter, peasants might be forced to consume foods that put their health further at risk.[21] Grains stored in damp indoor areas were prone to proliferation of the ergot fungus, which is poisonous when eaten. It attacks the muscular and circulatory systems, causing painful spasms and impaired blood flow to the extremities, which can lead to paralysis. It can also affect the brain, producing hallucinations and erratic behavior, and can eventually be fatal.[22]

Compounding this misery was the fact that, at least until the fifteenth century, the agricultural economy in which most people lived was local.[23] There were no reliable systems for shipping surplus goods from one region to another that was experiencing shortage.[24] Nor were there reliable ways to preserve foodstuffs, except by drying and salting them.[25] In times of need people might be forced to consume the fodder they had set aside for animals—meaning that the livestock would starve or have to be slaughtered for food.

Daily life during the long winters was especially harsh. Cold weather forced people indoors to spend the long hours of darkness huddled around whatever sources of heat they could find. The typical peasant's hovel consisted of one or two rooms, one with an open hearth for heat, and an inner chamber for sleeping and storage. There were few windows to let in light, and those were small and unglazed. The rooms were unventilated, unsanitary, cold, and damp. More fortunate people lived in longhouses, so called because they accommodated animals and family members under one roof but at opposite ends of the building. In the homes of the less fortunate, swine, cattle, and other farm animals were brought indoors to protect them from the elements. In most cases, houses had floors of mud, loosely covered with straw or rushes, or cobblestones. Houses were subject to flooding and chronically damp and moldy. The open hearth was an inefficient source of heat and poorly vented. The thin walls of the houses made them highly permeable to wind and weather. Rats were a constant menace, feeding on grain stored inside the house. Bathing and laundering under these conditions were virtually impossible, and the typical winter diet—salted meat and fish, bread made from coarse, poor-quality grains, and watery ale—virtually guaranteed illnesses caused by dietary deficiencies, infectious agents, and indigestible or toxic foods.[26]

Urban Living

Given the challenges of eking out a living by farming, some were forced or tempted to move to an urban area, but they could expect to find little relief or improvement in living standards there. Instead, town dwellers faced many of the challenges characteristic of life in the country, along with others. During the medieval period, only about a tenth of the population lived in urban settlements (with a population of two thousand or more).[27] The typical medieval urban environment was a toxic mix of filth, noise, rats, flies, and the terrible stench emanating from streets filled with raw sewage and garbage.[28] In the beginning stages of urban development in the tenth century, town dwellers typically lived on plots of land about a quarter or half an acre in size, with room to build houses and outbuildings and to plant gardens. But because most medieval towns were enclosed within city walls, as urban populations grew, the towns soon become overcrowded.[29] As peasants migrated to towns, lots were subdivided, so that by the twelfth century, people were often living in suffocating proximity to one another. Living quarters were placed adjacent to privies, or next to butchers' shops where animal entrails were simply dumped out onto the street, next to mounds of manure. Water supplies were polluted by sewage from privies running into open drains, contributing to the spread of dysentery.[30] As those who have studied urban life during the Middle Ages are fond of pointing out, the only real sanitation laws involved ordinances requiring homeowners to shout, "Look out below!" three times before emptying chamber pots out of their windows and onto the streets.[31]

These urban environments were breeding grounds for diseases of every kind. Archeological analyses of the contents of cesspits in urban areas show high concentrations of intestinal parasites, and though epidemic diseases could strike anywhere, in towns they could spread more rapidly and with far more devastating effects than in rural areas.[32]

Urban dwellers' diets were much like those of rural subsistence farmers. Bread and watery ale were the dietary staples, perhaps supplemented with milk, eggs, and fish. However, fish was scarce in inland areas, and during the winter months the low quality of feed available for livestock led to a progressive decline in concentrations of vitamin A available from milk and eggs.[33] In urban areas, regardless of season, certain foods, milk especially, were difficult to obtain and impossible to store for long periods. The winter diet of the average medieval citizen was essentially devoid of fruits and vegetables, except perhaps for small crops of carrots and cabbages that helped alleviate vitamin deficiencies; even then, the acreage available for such crops was small, and yields were poor. Not surprisingly, illnesses associated with vitamin deficiencies were endemic.

Life Expectancy

Under these nutritional and sanitary conditions in rural and urban areas, death was omnipresent.[34] It is difficult to state with precision the life expectancy of someone who had survived childhood, but a reasonable guess is that those who managed to remain alive until the age of twenty-five might survive into their early fifties.[35] One source states that although "evidence for infant mortality in the medieval countryside is wholly lacking. . . . [i]t is almost inconceivable that rates of infant mortality in the late Middle Ages were low, and . . . life expectancy at birth was less than thirty-five years, possibly less than thirty years."[36] One reliable source estimates that in the early fourteenth century, life expectancy at birth may have been as low as twenty-five.[37]

Many children died in early childhood. Some authorities estimate that more than one-third of all infants born during the Middle Ages died before reaching the age of five.[38] By comparison, infant mortality (death in the first twelve months of life) for 2005 in the United States was 29.4 per 100,000 live births.[39] Infants died from an array of conditions we would know today as influenza, respiratory diseases, whooping cough, measles, smallpox, accidents, tuberculosis, rashes, dehydration, urinary tract disorders, infections of the stomach and bowel, kidney stones, tumors and swellings of various kinds, hernias, ulcers, carbuncles, sores that would not heal, bone diseases, epilepsy, and even toothaches.[40]

When these high infant mortality rates are combined with deaths among the rest of the population, the result is a very short average life expectancy. According to Carole Rawcliffe, in Florence in the late 1420s life expectancy among laypeople was 29.5 years for women and 28.5 years for men.[41]

Death rates varied among different segments of the population. Those living in urban settlements were at greater risk of premature death. Excavations of urban cemeteries provide vivid evidence of the short and uncomfortable lives of urban dwellers. One such study found that 36 percent of men and 56 percent of women living in urban areas died before age thirty-five, and that only 9 percent of people lived to age sixty or later.[42] Examinations of skeletal remains find extensive evidence of malnutrition.[43] Archeological excavations of one medieval cemetery, St. Nicholas Shambles in London, produced 234 skeletons dating from the eleventh and twelfth centuries. Of the individuals whose bodies were exhumed, 94 percent had died before reaching the age of forty-five.[44] Other studies point to a variety of other kinds of illnesses, including typhoid fever, smallpox, cholera, malaria, tuberculosis, and dysentery.[45] Skeletal remains show signs of crippling rheumatism and poor dental health.

Those who sought escape in the quietude of a monastery in fact faced even higher odds of dying prematurely. According to one source, a young adult (age 16–20) who joined the monastic order at Westminster Abbey could expect to survive for only about ten years.[46] Between 1395 and 1505, the monastery at Canterbury experienced a major crisis in mortality on average every four years.[47] John Hatcher's study of the monks of Durham Priory in the years 1395–1529 shows similarly high mortality rates.[48] During outbreaks of the plague, mortality rates in monasteries were astronomically high. Among those who entered the Dominican monastery at Montpellier in France in 1347, only 5 percent of the monks in residence survived the plague of 1347–51; and in the Franciscan convents of Carcassonne and Marseille, every member of the community died.[49]

These high mortality rates continued well into the early modern period. The population of London at the beginning of the sixteenth century was in the range of fifty thousand. The annual mortality for this period has been estimated at five thousand per year, or about 10 percent of the entire population.[50] One study of birth and death records from London for the 1662 by the seventeenth-century English demographer John Gaunt finds that for every 100 live births, 60 children died before the age of sixteen, 36 of them during the first six years of life.[51] Not until the middle of the eighteenth century did life expectancy began to increase.

Common Illnesses

Among people of the medieval period, a sense of complete physical well-being was probably rare; most people probably suffered from multiple chronic diseases or disorders. Some kinds of illness can now be traced to vitamin deficiency. For example, one effect of vitamin A deficiency is a condition once termed "dry eyes," known today as xerophthalmia. In its early stages it causes night blindness, an inability to see in dim light. This disorder is the result of a failure of the tear glands to function properly. Night blindness put people at great risk of accidents.[52] Vitamin A deficiency can also cause conjunctivitis, an inflammation of the membranes that line the eyelids; painful bladder stones and urinary tract infections, both regularly reported among premodern populations; and diminished resistance to infections, often causing skin lesions.[53]

Shortages of meat, green vegetables, and fresh fruits, especially during the winter months, resulted in a serious vitamin C deficiency, which manifests itself as scurvy, causing chronic tiredness, muscle weakness, joint and muscle pain, rashes, and bleeding gums. Niacin deficiencies caused pellagra. Known today as the "disease of the four Ds," it causes diarrhea, dermatitis, dementia, and, if untreated, death. Those fortunate enough to escape pellagra were prone to develop other symptoms associated with niacin deficiency, such as ulcers of the mouth, nausea, vomiting, seizures, and disorders of balance. Vitamin D deficiency led to rickets in children. Parasites, such as lice and bed bugs, spread various diseases, some fatal.

Even a partial list of the diseases mentioned by historians of medieval medicine underscores how widespread disease-related morbidity would have been. In addition to plague, the list includes intestinal and pulmonary infections, typhus, and measles; sicknesses arising from malnutrition; mental and nervous disorders; leprosy, skin infections, smallpox, dropsy (edema), abscesses, and tumors of the liver; syphilis, tuberculosis, quinsy (tonsillitis), "pin and web" (an eye disease), fever, loss of hair, headaches, earaches, toothaches, nosebleeds, fainting spells, nausea, diarrhea, stomachaches, hemorrhoids, arthritis, and worms; and diseases of the spleen, chest, lungs, and urinary tract.[54]

These and other conditions were common among the population at large. Other diseases were associated with particular trades. The peasant who left the farmstead to mine coal risked developing black lung disease. Those who mined mercury faced a high risk of mercury poisoning. Becoming a metalsmith meant inhaling highly toxic vapors; becoming a potter meant exposure to lead poisoning. If the new line of work involved exposure to sulfur, workers would suffer the coughs and eye conditions associated with inhaling its fumes. Tanners were prone to develop dropsy from inhaling toxic fumes, and those who worked with glass were at risk of developing diseases of the chest.[55]

Famine and Plague

To the illnesses associated with chronic malnutrition, poor sanitation, and dangerous working conditions, nature added famine and deadly epidemics. The early 1300s saw the arrival of a cooling period in the earth's climate, which led to centuries of unsettled weather and much lower average temperatures throughout Europe.[56] One of the early consequences was the great famine of 1315–22, an event documented in riveting detail by William Jordan in his book *The Great Famine.* Jordan describes a seven-year period of extremely high rainfall: during one stretch it rained nonstop for 150 consecutive days throughout Western Europe.[57] The incessant rains made planting next to impossible, and the few crops that farmers managed to put into the ground could not be harvested because of flooding. Valuable topsoil washed away, as did salt basins, thereby depriving people of one of the few dependable methods for preserving food for the long winters. Food supplies were rapidly exhausted, leaving people to survive on tree bark, bird dung, family pets, and mildewed wheat and corn. These were interspersed with seven consecutive years of exceptionally cold winter weather, during which the North Sea twice froze over.

It is estimated that a half a million people (one in eight citizens) died in England during the Great Famine and that an estimated 10 to 15 percent of the urban population of Flanders and Germany perished. A large but unknowable proportion of the population of rural Europe succumbed as well.[58] In addition, the immune systems of those surviving on starvation diets were severely compromised, leaving them all but defenseless against disease.

Famine brought with it epidemics—typhoid fever, malaria, typhus, dysentery, and other gastrointestinal infections, smallpox, mumps, influenza, and, most deadly of all, plague. According to Carlo Cipolla, from 1346, when the first major plague epidemic occurred, until the end of the seventeenth century, scarcely a year went by without a large city or region of Europe reporting an epidemic of some kind.[59] Epidemics were not new, but earlier outbreaks of disease had had less devastating effects because of the lower population densities. The population growth that occurred before the cooling period, which allowed for the wider cultivation of land, paved the way for epidemics of devastating proportions. In some places, such as in England, the plague killed 35 to 40 of every 100 residents.[60]

Though no one understood at the time how the disease was transmitted, plague is caused by a bacterium, *Yersenia pestis*, carried by fleas whose preferred host is the rat.[61] Rats developed a natural tolerance to this bacillus that humans did not share. Plague takes three forms: bubonic, pneumonic, and septicemic. Bubonic plague attacks the lymph glands, causing painful swellings (termed *buboes*) all over the body, but mainly in the armpits and crotch. Death rates from the bubonic version of plague in the Middle Ages were high: 70 to 80 percent of those who became infected died in four to seven days.[62]

The pneumonic and septicemic strains of plague were deadlier still. Pneumonic plague is highly contagious. The lungs quickly fill with fluid, and victims can transmit the disease to other people by sneezing or spitting. In septicemic plague, the pathogen produces toxins that enter the bloodstream and produce a deep discoloration of the skin. This is one reason plague became known as the "Black Death."[63]

Plague caused not only great physical suffering and death but also economic and social disruption. Cipolla provides one especially graphic account of the chaos a plague epidemic could cause in his compelling monograph about the small Tuscan village of Monte Lupo.[64]

The plague first came to Monte Lupo in September 1630. When the health authorities in Florence were notified, they created a special cemetery outside the village walls. In addition, a pesthouse was built for the sick outside the village gate. Inside the village, quarantine was imposed on the households of victims. Those who were quarantined had to be fed, and this required the imposition of a special tax. Monte Lupo was already a very poor village, and its residents resisted the new tax. Civil unrest developed, exacerbated by the fact that thieves began to pillage

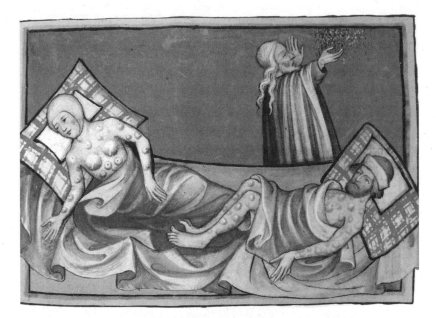

Figure 1. Victims of the Black Death. From the Toggenburg Bible, Switzerland, ca. 1411. Kupferstichkabinett, Staatliche Museen zu Berlin.

the abandoned households of some of the plague victims who had been sent to the pesthouse.

The epidemic continued to spread, so that by the beginning of 1631 the health magistracy in Florence proposed a general quarantine, attempting to confine the entire population of the village to their homes for a period of forty days.[65] Because such a measure threatened to cause the collapse of the local economy, tensions between the general populace and health officials escalated further.

At this point a serious conflict erupted between the health authorities, who favored quarantine, and a local priest, who believed that the only way to save the village was by appealing to God.[66] The priest announced his intention to parade the local parish church's most valuable relic—a crucifix—in a procession through the village. He invited the village congregation to join him, along with residents of nearby

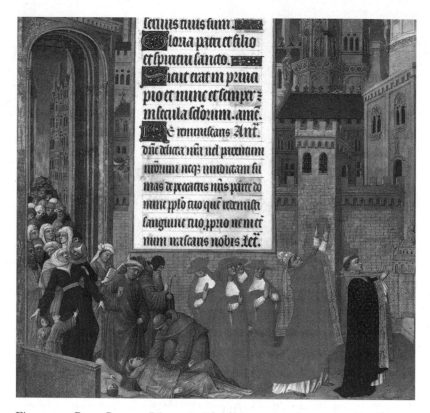

Figure 2.   Pope Gregory I (590–604) leading a procession to pray for the end of the plague in Rome. From *Les très riches heures du duc de Berry,* fifteenth century. Musée Condé, Chantilly. Courtesy of Art and Architecture Library, Stanford University.

communities that were also affected by the plague.[67] To enable these outsiders to join the procession, the priest's local supporters, under cover of darkness, dismantled the barrier that health officials had erected at the village gate. Outsiders poured into the village, and the villagers spread into the adjacent countryside. On the day of the procession, the church quickly filled with worshippers, and a vast procession made its way through the village, ending in the town square for a communal feast.

These events put health authorities completely at odds with the church and allowed the plague to spread throughout the village and the adjoining countryside. They also, of course, greatly worsened the already precarious economic and social state of Monte Lupo, so that in the end the plague not only caused widespread death but also effectively destroyed the social fabric of the community.

The Black Death tore at communal bonds in other ways, too. In *The Black Death*, based on sound historical scholarship, John Hatcher imaginatively reconstructs life in the medieval English village of Walsham in Suffolk. Hatcher describes the growing rifts between neighbors, the shunning of one another lest they themselves become infected, the warning away and barring of strangers from other villages, the unwillingness of those who were well to look after those who became ill, the inability or unwillingness of priests to perform customary burial rites, and the need to dispose of the dead by tossing them into open fields, ditches, and streams and rivers because of a shortage of consecrated burial space.[68]

This devastation of the existing social order did not end when the plague abated. The high death toll created an acute labor shortage, resulting in widespread neglect of established farmland, rising wages among the laboring classes, and a redistribution of wealth because the death of heirs transferred ownership of land to those who previously had none. Nor were the effects limited to economic arrangements. The plague insidiously eroded beliefs among survivors in religious doctrines and those who preached them. Ordinary people had been told that the plague was God's revenge for their sins and that to stop the Black Death they needed to confess them fully. Hatcher explains: "Walsham's inhabitants, like people everywhere and in all ages, argued, lied, cheated, stole, and fornicated; they reneged on debts, charged exorbitant rates of interest, misrepresented the quality and quantity of goods they sold and falsely denigrated those they bought, repeatedly cut their lords' and their neighbors' hedges for firewood, encroached on the property of others and carelessly or maliciously allowed their cows, sheep, pigs and geese to stray." This meant that there was much to confess, and the evidence Hatcher cites suggests that people owned up to their failings out of fear of continuing divine vengeance. Yet no matter how hard they prayed and how often they confessed, the deaths continued, leaving many of the faithful survivors wondering why God should react so angrily to minor misdeeds.[69] In the end, they lost confidence in the explanation their priests had given them for the plague. Moreover, because of the high death rates among the priesthood, the people lost faith in their priests as spiritual brokers favored by God.

Accidents, Fire, and Violence

If poor diet, dreadful sanitation, famine, and epidemics contributed to appallingly high rates of premature death, so too did accidents. In the United States today, the overall death rate from accidents is estimated to be 40.6 per 100,000 population.[70] Although no comparable figures exist for the communities of medieval Europe, these were very dangerous places, and accidents were common. Children were expected to contribute to the household economy by fishing and drawing water, and some of them drowned while performing these tasks.[71] Tiny infants and toddlers were often left unattended for long periods during the day while their parents worked, and, as Carol Rawcliffe explains, "the juxtaposition in dark, cramped surroundings of open hearths, straw bedding, rush-covered floors and naked flames posed a constant threat to curious infants." Even at play, "children were in danger because of ponds, agricultural or industrial implements, stacks of timber, unattended boats and loaded wagons, all of which appear with depressing frequency in coroners' reports as causes of death among the young. Besides the obvious risk to health presented by the close proximity of domestic animals, which either shared their owner's quarters or wandered in off the streets, the very real possibility that one would maim or kill a child increased the odds against survival even more."[72]

Those who lived in rural settlements faced other hazards. In his book *At Day's Close*, Roger Ekirch describes the environment in which most people lived: "Much of the pre-industrial landscape remained

treacherous. . . . Steep hillsides, turbulent streams, and thick under-
brush cut across pastures, fields and villages. Even when lands had been
cleared in Europe by agriculture, tree stumps and trenches scarred the
rock-strewn terrain. Thick slabs of peat, cut for fuel, left deep ditches.
In parts of England, Wales and Scotland with active or abandoned col-
lieries, quarries and coal-pits pocked the ground."[73] The combination of
the endemic night blindness due to dietary deficiencies and the absence
of artificial light meant that nighttime heightened the dangers posed by
these hazards. Those unfortunate or foolish enough to venture out after
dark were in constant danger of falling into an open ditch, pond, or river;
man-made hazards included wells, moats, canals, and, worst of all, cess-
pools. There were discarded tree stumps to avoid, plow furrows and ruts
to trip into. And because of the darkness, it was easy to lose one's way.

Barbara Hanawalt, who has creatively analyzed the records of formal
inquests of unexpected deaths for this period, shows the pervasiveness of
accidental deaths, especially drownings. For patrons of local alehouses,
inebriation made the journey home that much more dangerous.[74]

Urban environments were just as hazardous. The great majority of
urban settlements were disorderly rabbit warrens of narrow streets and
alleys, crammed with small houses. Until the second half of the seventeenth century, when street lamps were introduced into the great cities
of Europe, the only sources of light in the streets were candles and oil
lamps shining through the windows of houses. Bands of thieves often
roamed at night; any urbanite who ventured out after dark put his life at
risk. In fact, Ekirch reports that the murder rate during the early modern era was five to ten times higher than today. According to one source,
homicides were twice as frequent as deaths from accidents, and only one
of every one hundred murderers was ever brought to justice.[75]

Some municipal institutions existed, but they closed before dark so
that workers could go home before nightfall. For protection at night, all
the residents could do was retreat inside their homes and secure them
with locks, bolts, shutters, and gates. For added protection, they were
advised to get a guard dog and to arm themselves.[76]

The extraordinary lengths to which some municipalities went to protect themselves from thieves, brigands, and others at night is illustrated by Ekirch's discussion of the French town of Saint-Malo, a garrison town on the northern coast of France that housed large quantities of naval stores. In the early 1600s, to discourage thievery, local authorities released packs of unfed mastiffs into the streets after dark to prowl for food. The animals roamed the streets all night and would set on any living thing on the streets after sundown.[77]

Fire posed an equal hazard. In rural areas, most homes had open hearths set in the middle of rooms built of tinder-dry wood, their floors covered with flammable straw, and their roofs made of thatch. Clothes left to dry hanging next to fireplaces were in danger of catching fire, as were chimneys clogged with soot. Candles and oil lamps could easily set fire to objects they touched.[78] Most agricultural settlements consisted of houses and barns arranged in close proximity. A fire ignited in any of these structures could easily spread to other buildings. The only means of fighting fire was with leather water buckets and hooks to pull timbers and straw from burning structures.

In urban areas, fire posed special dangers. The tinderbox structures that were homes to the urban poor were crammed together into congested rows, so that a fire breaking out in any one of them could spread quickly to consume entire blocks of houses and even the entire settlement. According to Ekirch, in England from 1500 to 1800, at least 421 fires in provincial towns consumed ten or more houses apiece, with as many as 46 fires during the period destroying one hundred or more houses. Some larger urban areas were all but consumed by great fires, including Toulouse in 1463, Bourges in 1487, and Troyes in 1534.[79]

Fear of God's Wrath

Added to this already toxic mix of elements was another, ironically supplied by the prevailing religious orthodoxy of the day. Religion offered comfort to the faithful, but it also injected a powerful sense of fear into everyday life.[80] The common conception of God was one of a vengeful, all-powerful, all-knowing being, an image that fostered a pervasive sense of fear and foreboding.[81] He controlled life from moment to moment: everything that happened, from the most banal events to the epic, were signs of his agency. The belief that an external force controlled daily life contributed to a kind of collective paranoia.[82] Rainstorms, thunder, lightning, wind gusts, solar or lunar eclipses, cold snaps, heat waves, dry spells, and earthquakes alike were considered signs and signals of God's displeasure. As a result, the "hobgoblins of fear" inhabited every realm of life. The sea became a satanic realm, and forests were populated with beasts of prey, ogres, witches, demons, and very real thieves and cutthroats. This aura of terror was pervasive. Ekirch writes: "At night, bizarre sights and queer sounds came and vanished, leaving widespread anxiety in their train." After dark, too, the world was filled with omens portending dangers of every sort: comets, meteors, shooting stars, lunar eclipses, the howls of wild animals.[83]

As if all the suffering caused by natural events were not enough, medieval people displayed a seemingly insatiable appetite for barbaric acts of violence.[84] They waged wars against one another, attacked neighboring villages and neighbors in their own communities, slaughtered heretics, burned witches, and visited acts of physical and sexual abuse on one another.[85] This problem of violence extended not just to neighbors arguing with neighbors, people from adjacent villages in dispute, or roving bans of brigands looting rural settlements. Rawcliffe, describing the practice of surgery during the Middle Ages, points out that "levels of domestic violence were so great that local surgeons became quite experienced at treating head wounds, internal injuries, broken bones and stab wounds."[86]

Historians generally agree that violence was endemic. Goodich writes: "The employment of violence as a means of dealing with conflict, however petty, had become a widely learned cultural trait."[87] Miller and Hatcher state that "men were swift to defend their rights by force and, when quarrels arose, to resort to the knife or other weapons" and that "excessive violence was characteristic of the epoch."[88] This violence extended to every aspect of medieval life, from personal disputes to group vendettas, from organized, illegitimate violence such as sea piracy to organized open warfare.[89]

What explains this readiness to resort to violence? Poverty was surely one factor. Poverty promotes crime, and high rates of crime in turn give rise to fear among potential victims. In the absence of a strong police force or other public bodies to provide protection or control retribution, medieval people were left to protect themselves, and one way to do this was to assault perceived sources of threat.[90] The ready availability of weapons, access to alcohol, the likelihood of escaping punishment, and the general ethos of violence all contributed to the toxic mix.

The medieval world was based on a culture of honor, expressed in the form of incessant demands for deference and respect.[91] Those who study such cultures tell us that they are also characterized by an ethos of individual power, masculinity, and self-protection.[92] To establish and preserve one's sense of honor, and to ensure self-protection, members learn to react violently to even subtle cues of insult and attack.[93] Research by the social psychologists Richard Nisbett and Dov Cohen has shown how this tendency is displayed in face-to-face relationships between members of communities, suggesting that cultures of honor are most likely to develop where no effective policing powers are available to protect individuals and their property.[94]

Finally, religion tended to foster violence. Throughout Europe, violence was routinely used to uncover and then punish heretics, and justified as necessary in the execution of God's work.[95]

Writing about the lifetime of the fourth-century saint Martin of Tours, the medievalist Raymond van Dam provides a characterization of those times that applies equally well to life during the later medieval and early modern periods. He describes a life that was "unrelentingly brutal and precarious . . . with squalor, misery, and grinding poverty . . . violence, cruelty, intemperate weather, locusts, a late frost, hailstorms, drought, poor nutrition, illnesses and disabilities."[96]

THE WEAKNESS OF CIVIC INSTITUTIONS

Today, in times of crisis, we turn almost automatically to public institutions, agencies, and services for help. But in medieval times there was no fire department to summon to a chimney fire, no police department to catch thieves, no ambulance to transport the sick. Also missing were sanitation services, a meaningful criminal-justice system, and a standing army to protect against invasion. Systems for controlling floods were not always effective; there was no provision for communal long-term storage of food as a guard against starvation, no water-purification system or reservoirs in which to store water, no protection against extreme weather. The most powerful secular figure was the king, yet in most cases even he could do little to help, and in any event he could intervene only where he was physically present; hence his protection was restricted to those who had direct access to him.[97] Even if the telephone had existed, a 911 number would have been useless. There was little or no help to be summoned.

Medieval Medicine

The institution of medicine was hopelessly ill-equipped to deal with the terrible tolls on health exacted by medieval living conditions. Practitioners of medicine consisted of a ragtag collection of barbers, herbalists, folk healers, astrologers, dentists, witches, and quacks. Any understanding of how and why people became ill or recovered was provided by the classical Greek notion of the four humors succinctly explained by Carol Rawcliffe: "Just as the universe was made up of the four basic elements of fire, water, earth and air, so too the body depended for its existence on four corresponding human humors created through the digestive process out of food: cholera or yellow bile; phlegm or mucus; black bile and blood." Good health required maintaining a careful balance between these and ensuring that none grew either too powerful or too weak.[98] Treatment consisted "in examining the patient, particularly the urine, and in diagnosing an imbalance of the four humours. . . . The imbalance could then be corrected by means of purges, bloodletting, special diets, and so forth."[99]

Such corrections entailed unpleasant, painful, and occasionally even fatal procedures. Patients were bled; heated glass vessels were placed on areas of skin that had been scarred with a knife; leeches were applied to open wounds to draw off poisons; patients were cauterized using caustic medicines or heated implements; and foul-smelling herbs, fumigants, and vile-tasting concoctions were administered by mouth or to the skin. Those diagnosed with demonic possession were flogged, beaten, starved, or, in effect, waterboarded. As if the pain caused by such treatments were not bad enough, the physician or surgeon sometimes took added steps. Many surgeons believed that the premature cleansing, drying, or closing of a wound would force corrupt matter inward and poison the patient.[100] Accordingly, after a procedure involving cauterization or scarring, the physician might bandage the wound with cotton that had been soaked in salt water to ensure that it did not heal too quickly.

Because bodily processes were linked with cosmic developments, the physician also consulted a patient's horoscope to understand the disposition of the heavens at the moment of his birth and at the time he became ill and to track the conjunction of the planets at each stage of treatment. This deeply held belief in the role of heavenly bodies in human illness occasionally gave rise to bizarre explanations for epidemics. For example, in 1348 Philip VI turned to the faculty of the University of Paris for an explanation of why the Black Death was sweeping his kingdom. The medical team reported that the outbreak of plague was beyond the ability of humans to control: it was caused by the conjunction of three planets in the sign of Aquarius, which, along with other conjunctions and eclipses, had produced a pernicious corruption of the air. They dated the cause of the epidemic to one o'clock on the afternoon of March 20, 1345, when the deadly alignment of heavenly bodies occurred.[101]

The same logic might lead physicians to propose that an illness could only be treated on certain days of the year. Those who were diagnosed with dropsy needed to undergo a regimen of bloodletting, but only on September 17. Migraine headaches needed to be treated on April 3, eye problems on April 11, and so on. If a patient sued a doctor for malpractice, the role of celestial bodies in causing illness could be used in deciding the case. One source describes a malpractice suit that was brought against three physicians in 1424 by a patient who had sought treatment for a wounded thumb. The case was thrown out on the grounds that the injury had occurred on the last day of January, a time when, as the medical specialists' report argued, "the moon was consumed with a bloody sign, to wit Aquarius, under a very malevolent constellation, and that, even worse, some nine days later, by which time the moon had passed into Gemini (the sign governing the hand . . .). In other words, the plaintiff could consider himself fortunate to have survived at all against such tremendous odds."[102]

Most medical care, however useless, was reserved for the rich.[103] As Faye Getz notes, "The pressing problems of famine, epidemic disease, and social dislocation among the poor made resort to medical practitioners nearly impossible."[104]

RELIGION AND COMMUNITY AS BUFFERS AGAINST ADVERSITY

The picture we have painted of life for the average European in the medieval period is bleak indeed, but it is incomplete. Fortunately, people seldom had to confront these grim conditions entirely alone. In normal times, two social institutions served as buffers against adversity, made life manageable and tolerable, and imbued it with a vital sense of meaning: religion and community. The two were intimately entwined, yet each made a distinctive contribution to the quality of daily life. From our vantage point in the twenty-first century, what they offered might not seem very effective, but to those who lived in medieval and early modern Europe, they must certainly have provided much-needed comfort and reassurance.

Living in agricultural communities of the sort I have described was a quintessentially communal existence. To survive, everyone had to accept a certain degree of regulation and offer mutual support. Christopher Dyer explains why: at the heart of communal life during this period "lay the management of the common land, especially when all of the arable in a midland field system was subject to common grazing. The pressure on land meant that rules had to be observed or neighbors would suffer." Regulations governed the planting and harvesting of crops, grazing rights, prohibited poaching, and encouraged people to look after one another. Everyone recognized their common interest in cooperating to keep agriculture running smoothly.[105] This is not to say that people never acted independently or that they lacked entrepreneurial skills, but only that the culture placed a high value on cohesive communality.

The need for everyone to work together to survive contributed to a powerful sense of community and a corresponding feeling of security and mutual support in adversity.[106] In performing the daily tasks of a small agricultural community, individuals were reminded at nearly every turn of the importance and value of the collective enterprise.

The term *community* in this context should not be taken to imply a single, overarching entity. Instead, it connotes clusters of memberships in different kinds of groups: households, neighborhoods, villages, parishes, guilds, and workshops, as well as counties, regions, and nation-states. These multiple associates made personal identity somewhat fluid, yet rooted in the security of embeddedness in a social world.[107]

Religious belief and practice powerfully reinforced this sense of community. Early modern Christian communities centered on the parish and its teachings: belief in God, Jesus Christ, and the Holy Ghost, as well as the obligation of parishioners to confess their sins, take communion, and attend mass. These articles of faith gave people a powerful sense of identification with the church at large, reminding us that, "even in the most remote of English farmsteads, there were tenets of belief which its inhabitants shared not only with neighboring villages but with villages as far afield as the Baltic and the Mediterranean."[108] Another historian writes:

"Religious life for Medieval Christians was predominantly a communal experience. They practiced their faith in the context of a parish, the basic unit of public worship: Where one lived determined what parish one belonged to, and within its boundaries, a medieval Christian learned his or her creed, received moral instruction and correction, received his sacraments and paid taxes, collected tithes to support the church. Communal life was both supportive and coercive, and much of the laity's parish involvement comprised balancing these two forces."[109]

In the local parish church, the faithful were instructed in the tenets of the Catholic faith and inducted into its practices. Phillipp Schofield explains:

> Throughout an individual's life, the union with the Church was maintained through the sacraments which, organized around vital moments in that life, reaffirmed a relationship with Church and God. Through the sacrament of baptism, a sacrament typically administered within hours of birth, the newborn were admitted into membership of the church while, at the point of death, the sacrament of extreme unction prepared the penitent for death and membership of a new congregation in the life everlasting. In between these two 'moments,' other sacraments strengthened the relationship between the church and the individual—the marriage rite . . . confession, the Eucharist, confirmation.[110]

Membership in a parish church entailed more than attending mass, communion, and confession. It also involved the obligation to support and maintain the church buildings and property and support its priest.[111] Church-sponsored confraternities were often organized in the name of a favorite saint. In times of need they fed the hungry, clothed the poor, provided dowries for needy young women, looked after the sick, and buried the dead. They also staged processions and met for private devotion. Thus membership in the parish church tightly integrated people into religious communities.[112]

William Christian has studied in impressive detail the role that religious belief and practice play in rural Spanish communities today. His study documents how religious doctrines infuse and structure family and community relationships, mirroring people's relationships with God, the Virgin, saints, and the Catholic Church, and how relationships with the divine in turn are patterned on family ties.[113]

The important role that religion played, and still plays, in helping buffer people against adversity was succinctly captured by the sociologist Émile Durkheim, who wrote in 1912: "The true function of religion is not to make us think. Its true function is to make us act and to help us live. The believer who has communed with his god is not simply a man who sees new truths that the unbeliever knows not; he is a man who is stronger within himself, he feels more strength to endure the trials of existence or to overcome them. He is as though lifted above the human miseries, because he is lifted above his human condition."[114]

Of all the features of medieval religion, the faith in saints was one of the most potent. Ordinary people thought of them as friends, protectors, advocates, and personal intercessors with God. It is not difficult to understand why. Given the inability of social institutions to protect or assist individuals, in particular the poor and powerless, the only line of defense against adversity was the agency of God and his saints.

The great challenge facing individuals and communities was devising ways of gaining access to these powers. The next chapter examines the actions people took to invite divine intervention into their lives and the beliefs that gave rise to these actions.

CHAPTER TWO

Saints

Yearning for divine protection and miracles, medieval people did not merely register their request with a saint and then stand by, waiting for good things to happen. Accounts of miracles always refer to some form of human activity undertaken in conjunction with requests made of saints—a prayer, an act of veneration, a confession, a pilgrimage, a presentation of gifts. These actions offered no guarantee of a miracle, but not engaging in them precluded any possibility of one.

Actions undertaken in the hope of inducing a miracle were not improvised but highly codified by the dictates of medieval culture and religion. This chapter explains the reasoning behind these practices. How did people think miracles came about? To whom should they turn to receive one? How should such a figure be approached? With what words and demeanor should an appeal be made? And what was the belief system on which these and related questions rested?

CONNECTIONS AMONG PEOPLE, SAINTS, AND GOD

Appeals for miracles from ordinary people were always addressed to divine actors in a grand drama. The script of this drama involved three sets of relationships: those of humans with God, of saints with God, and of saints with humans. The role of saints in facilitating miracles was constructed by beliefs about the other two groups of actors and the relationships between them.

Humans' Relationships with God

A paradox lay at the heart of the drama. Although people believed that God was the sole source of miracles, they addressed their appeals for miracles to saints.[1] One explanation of this paradox can be found in the image ordinary people held of God and the implications this image had for the possibility—or, more accurately, the impossibility—of relating to and addressing appeals directly to him. Approaching him head-on, so to speak, was a prospect too terrifying to contemplate. People needed to devise other, indirect ways to gain his attention.

Religious doctrine portrayed God as an all-powerful, incorporeal being, the mightiest of imaginable forces—beyond history, immanent in the world, a formless, anonymous, eternal, disembodied, luminous essence that was nowhere in particular yet everywhere at once and forever, a distant and severe power, quick to anger.[2] What possible reason would such a force have for even noticing human supplicants, much less heeding their pleas? Moreover, God was the final arbiter of human events. If a direct appeal to him went unheeded, it might spell the end of all hope.

People ascribed to the saints qualities that made them ideal candidates for mediating requests for miracles. To understand what these qualities are and how saints came to acquire them, we need to understand the relationships between saints and God.

Saints' Relationships with God

According to the medieval way of thinking, saints held special sway with God.[3] Their influence with him came about through actions that had led God to accord them a special state of grace (*sanctus*).[4] Most writings about saints—hagiographies, martyrologies, religious tracts, and so on—recount how and why these particular people attained this standing. For example, the apostles, the evangelists, and figures such as the Virgin Mary acquired *sanctus* because of their roles in Christ's life.[5] Others attained *sanctus* through martyrdom, having been put to death for proclaiming their faith at times and places where Christianity was outlawed. Because of their suffering on behalf of the faith, they were said to enjoy a special intimacy with God.[6] In A.D. 313, in the Edict of Milan, the Roman emperor Constantine legalized Christianity, and subsequently the practice of martyrdom became less common. As martyrs diminished in number, they were succeeded by "confessors"—bishops, other clergy, monks, nuns, and laypersons whose lives demonstrated a heroic faith and integrity.[7] Later still came those who were accorded the status of saint either by the acclamation of local citizens or by the actions of the local bishop, or sometimes by both.[8] On dying, it was believed, saints ascended directly to heaven and sat at the feet of God.

From this position of intimacy, saints were well positioned to intercede for individuals on earth. God would grant a supplicant's wish not because of the person's virtues but out of his admiration for the saint to whom the request was made. As one authority explains it: "It was as if the servants of God had acquired, through the sufferings they had endured during their lifetime, a means of putting pressure on God, in a sense obliging him to intervene on behalf of whoever had put themselves under their protection."[9] Another authority adds: "The saint, connected with higher powers, employed his magical capabilities to help his worshippers, easing their lives, healing their illnesses, averting natural or social calamities, freeing the unfortunate and the powerless from oppression. In return, the saint required obedience, veneration, and gifts for the church founded under his patronage."[10]

Because of their closeness to God, saints were also presumed to know better than ordinary people how best to approach and relate to him. In addition, having once dwelled among the living, saints were viewed as figures who could understand and sympathize with human needs and imperfections in a way that an angry and brooding God did not.

All of the powers ascribed to the "ordinary" dead, of course, extended to saints as well, but, to draw on Peter Brown's apt characterization, saints were "the Very Special Dead" and were endowed with additional powers and attributes.[11] When ordinary people died, their bodies were believed to remain on earth to decay; their souls, which departed the body at the moment of death, went to purgatory (or if they had been truly evil, directly to hell). For saints, things were different. Their souls ascended directly to heaven, but their being also remained attached to their physical remains on earth. Thus a saint had a presence in this world as well as in heaven and could exercise influence in both.

Humans' Relationships with Saints

Saints, then, enjoyed special agency and moved freely between heaven and earth. The cult of saints, to quote Brown, was thus about "the joining of Heaven and Earth, and the role, in this joining, of dead human beings." Their graves became "privileged places, where the contrasted poles of heaven and Earth met."[12]

In Brown's words, saints were "approachable" and understandable, whereas God was not. He explains that saints personalized the worship of God by providing people with what he terms an "intimate invisible friend."[13] In their relationships with saints, ordinary people employed the same principles and strategies that governed everyday human associations. They devised ways to curry favor with the saints to persuade them to intercede for them with God. And appealing to a saint offered an advantage that a direct appeal to God did not. If, following an appeal to a saint, a miracle did not happen, this did not signal the end of all hope. One could appeal to the saint a second time, or, because saints were numerous, simply direct the request to another.

Saints, moreover, were regarded as present in the earthly world. In his fascinating book *Living with the Dead in the Middle Ages*, Patrick Geary explains that the dead were regarded as active members of the community, beings who retained a presence in human affairs.[14] Though invisible, they were considered friends, sources of protection, inspiration, and solace.[15] It also seemed logical to assume that saints would observe the rules that governed social relationships among the living. One of the most fundamental of these was reciprocity—the expectation that gifts given would be reciprocated. Aron Gurevich explains: "The principle of 'a gift ought to be rewarded' was one of the basic principles of social relations in barbarian and early feudal society and it . . . extended to relations between laymen and saints."[16] Thus leaving coins and other valuables at the place where the saint's relics lay in repose created an obligation for the saint to reciprocate. Of course, most donors probably would not have thought of gifts to saints in quite so instrumental a way. To them, gifts were viewed primarily as expressions of their admiration and love for the saint. But at the heart of this practice lay the hope that by accepting the gift, the saint would be honor-bound to reciprocate by arranging a miracle.

For this reason, most requests for a miraculous cure were coupled with a gift to the saint. William Christian explains that the offerings varied:

> Working for a certain number of days on the shrine construction, sending workers, lime, stone, or wood; or other traditional Mediterranean votive offering such as money, figures in wax of eyes, tongues, hands, faces, or entire bodies; a wax model of a cured horse or wax symbols of captivity, such as chains or manacles. People spared from death or raised from the dead sent or brought shrouds, the crosses of wax with which they were laid out, and other funeral paraphernalia. People offered their own physical penances—coming barefoot or on their knees. . . . At the shrine they might spend the night praying or even staying for nine days of novena.[17]

These practices explain why the shrines of popular saints could become such important sources of wealth for cathedrals and churches. The inventory of objects deposited at famous shrines is little short of astounding. They included coins, bread, wine, jewelry, fowl, grains, fruits and vegetables, livestock, cloth, precious metals, clothing, tools, and household goods. Quantities of wax, highly valued for making candles to illuminate the interiors of churches, were often contributed as well. According to the custom of the day, gifts of wax should be the same size as the donor's body or, if accompanying appeals for the healing of a particular body part, the same weight and length as the afflicted limb or organ.

In his monumental study *Sainthood in the Later Middle Ages,* André Vauchez presents the following inventory of items found at Hereford Cathedral's tomb of Thomas of Cantilupe: "170 silver ships, 41 wax ships, 129 silver images of a person or of human limbs, 1,424 wax images of a person or of human limbs, 77 animal figures, 108 crutches, and 3 wooden vehicles."[18] Jonathan Sumption cites an entry by an eleventh-century chronicler at Saint Christina's shrine in Saint-Trond near Liège, Belgium, that listed "herds of animals . . . palfreys [saddled horses], cows and bulls, pigs, lambs, and sheep. Linen, wax, bread, and cheese arrived; and above all purses of money." So much money was given that several men were needed to collect it in the evening and put it in a safe place, and a number of monks worked full-time as guardians of the shrine.[19]

Giving gifts, of course, offered no guarantee of a miracle. All one could do was give and ask; it was up to the saint to decide whether to appeal to God on the supplicant's behalf, and then up to God to decide whether to act. In this sense, giving gifts to a saint was analogous to buying a lottery ticket today: buying a ticket does not guarantee a win, but without a ticket one has no chance at all.

APPEALING TO SAINTS FOR MIRACLES

Selecting, approaching, and addressing saints were complex matters requiring elaborate preparatory steps. The supplicant had to place herself in a proper frame of mind and abide by strict codes of conduct involving dress, posture, language, and general demeanor.

Choosing the Right Saint

People first had to decide which saint to appeal to. In some circumstances, of course, one might have no real choice. In isolated areas, the only accessible saint might be the patron of the village. Poverty or other circumstances might preclude a pilgrimage to a distant shrine to venerate a particular saint.[20] Where choices existed, the supplicant might follow the example of some and decide by lottery, for example by "seeing which . . . saint's name was drawn three times from a bag."[21] Such outcomes were sometimes interpreted as signs from the saints.

One basis for choosing which saint to appeal to was the nature of the miracle desired. By the thirteenth century, Christianity boasted a vast array of saints who specialized in facilitating miracles of different kinds.[22] Certain saints gained renown for curing blindness, rickets, arthritis, or madness. Others were famous for their ability to avert or end drought, prevent violence, or protect people against fire. For relief from the plague one might be advised to turn to Saint Roch or Saint Sebastian. If you were suffering from the pox, Saint Job was your best choice. For relief from botches and boils, you might appeal to Saint Cosmus or Saint Damian. Saint Clare was said to specialize in curing disorders of the eyes, Saint Apollonia cured toothaches, Saint Oswald and Saint Faith worked miracle cures with animals, and so on.[23] Just as today we consult the proper medical specialists for help with our ailments, so too medieval people approached the saint with the best reputation for facilitating cures for a specific condition.

To win favor with a saint, it was vital to demonstrate personal loyalty. To venerate a number of saints promiscuously in hopes that a miracle would occur through the actions of one of them, or to turn to just any saint regardless of specialty, might cause offense. The supplicant also had to consider a saint's position in the celestial pecking order. In thirteenth-century Christianity, those who dwelled in heaven were imagined to form a pyramid-shaped hierarchy. Christ stood at the apex, and immediately below him the Virgin Mary. Then came the apostles,

John the Baptist, and later a few of the most renowned saints, such as Saint Francis of Assisi, Saint Anthony of Padua, and Saint Isidore of Seville. At the bottom of the pyramid were the humblest saints, known only to members of a particular village or perhaps only to a single family. Between the apex and the base dwelled hundreds of others revered for their good deeds, including martyrs, church officials of every rank, prophets, and seers.

The rules that applied to relationships between ordinary people and saints were also believed to apply to relationships between saints. The lower a saint's place in the hierarchy, the more levels their appeals needed to negotiate before reaching the ear of God. Certain saints were considered to occupy especially strategic places in heaven, whereas lesser saints, such as local patron saints, could appeal to God's influence only through the more influential saints above them. People therefore attempted to appeal to the most influential saint they could, not only because these saints were believed to have more direct and greater influence with God but also because the more numerous the levels through which the appeal had to ascend, the greater the complexity of reciprocal obligations and the greater the risk of distorting or misrepresenting the message.

Some preferred to appeal not to saints who had already been canonized but instead to what were thought of as saints-in-waiting. The reasoning was that the potential payoff could be huge. People imagined saints-in-waiting to be more responsive to appeals for miracle cures as a way of establishing their own credentials for sainthood, and they were less likely to be inundated with appeals.[24] Such tactics were not without risks, of course, as supplicants might well be directing their requests for miracle cures to figures whose special status was unproven.

Approaching the Saint

Though in practice saints could be venerated anywhere, they were thought to be most responsive to prayers offered near the place where their relics lay in repose, or where their apparitions had been seen.

Although resident in Heaven, the saint was also believed to be present at his tomb on earth.[25] The optimal time to visit the saint's tomb or hallowed space was on his feast day.[26]

A person's relationship to the saints, then, was patterned on the principles that governed relations with other people. The same rules of reciprocity applied, as did the strategies for gaining favor with those higher in status and the methods of promoting one's case with authority figures.

Because saints were believed to be present both in heaven and on earth, they were frequently endowed with very human qualities. Ronald Finucane recounts how the saint William of Norwich reportedly appeared to an admirer in a vision to express his anger about pilgrims soiling his tomb with spittle. A young Norwich girl described a vision in which William complained of having developed a stiff neck from lying awkwardly in his coffin. An admirer of the saint Edmund Rich claimed that he had had a dream in which the saint reported that he could no longer work miracles because the earth over his tomb was so heavy that he was unable to raise his hands to assist supplicants. Saint Godric of Finchale reportedly confided to a dreamer his aversion to the stench of the public latrines near the church where he was buried. Other pilgrims reported dreams and visions in which they saw the saints lift their coffin's lid to get in and out. A famous window of Canterbury Cathedral depicts Saint Thomas Becket floating out of his tomb.[27] There is also the example of a Frankish king who prayed to Martin of Tours for permission to remove the body of the king's enemy from the church where Martin's relics lay. A blank piece of parchment was left on Martin's tomb for three days in anticipation of a reply. When no answer appeared on it, the king accepted that Martin had denied his request.[28]

Through their dual presence in this world and the next, saints could bring the powers of heaven to bear on events and people on earth. This power was exercised through holy relics: pieces of bone, strands of hair, finger- and toenail clippings, teeth, fragments of clothing, pieces of shoes—any actual body parts or material objects that had come into direct contact with a saint's body.[29]

The Significance of Relics

Saints' relics made it possible for the devout to connect with saints. They were objects that one could see, before which one could kneel and pray, and to which one could present gifts. They were thought of as "still heavy with the fullness of a beloved person" and imbued with qualities that made them conduits for miraculous forces.[30] In the language of present-day epidemiology, relics were regarded as the vectors by which miracles granted by God were transmitted through the saint to the body of an individual or to a community.

Relics lay at the heart of the medieval cult of saints. One historian asserts: "The true religion of the Middle Ages . . . is the worship of relics. . . . To the masses religion was the veneration of the remains of saints or of objects that had been used by Jesus or the Virgin. It was believed that divine intervention in human affairs manifested itself . . . through the power of relics."[31] Geary explains: "Relics were the main channel through which supernatural power was available for the needs of ordinary life. Ordinary men could see and handle them, yet they belonged not to this transitory world but to eternity. . . . Among all the objects of the visible, malign, unintelligible world, relics were both visible and full of beneficent intelligence." Elsewhere the same author flatly asserts: "The relics were the saint."[32]

This idea, that the relic and saint were one and the same, will be familiar to students of object and agency, a concept that is gaining currency in social science. It focuses on an idea initially put forward by the French sociologist Émile Durkheim in *The Elementary Forms of Religious Life*. Durkheim focused on the role of sacred objects in totemic religions. He was interested in the way totems—pieces of stone and wood—became sacred objects, material things that the sacred force was believed to inhabit.[33] People seem to find it easier to relate to forces like the sacred by creating concrete material objects that represent sacredness, and then granting agency to these objects to affect human events. A strand of hair belonging to a saint becomes the saint's embodiment, so that touching, feeling, and seeing the hair itself is necessary to experience the saint's power.[34] The relics of saints are prime examples of the phenomenon of object and agency in action.

A saint's relics were imbued with a special force: *virtus*, a quality conferred by God on saints alone, whose presence was revealed by a number of distinct physiological signs.[35] One was the incorruptibility of the saint's flesh. Vauchez explains: "It was believed that the mortal remains of the saints did not experience the same fate as those of ordinary mortals. Once life had gone out of their body, it became 'soft as the flesh of a child,' which was a first sign of their divine election. Before being laid in the ground, the body remained in this state for many days, so that the dead person seemed to be sleeping rather than dead. Once buried, the body was supposed not to decompose." Another was the so-called "odor of sanctity," the sweet and pleasant odor given off by the body of someone whom God had anointed a saint.[36]

Virtus infused a saint's soul and bodily remains as well as any objects with which the saint had direct physical contact. The force was believed to be present in the saint's clothing, in the tomb, in the soil that surrounded the tomb, in the liquids that oozed from it, and in anything else that had been in immediate or near contact with the saint's body. Saints' relics thus suffused with *virtus* were treated as if surrounded by a force field of spirituality, what one scholar has aptly termed "holy radioactivity."[37] This emanation, which could be transmitted to anyone who came near it, served as the medium for the saint's miraculous powers to heal.

To experience the full strength and benefits of this force, pilgrims believed that they should get as close to the relic as physically possible. Thus, the most desirable way to venerate a saint was to go to the tomb or the site of the saint's relics and get as close to them as possible. The point of visiting a saint's tomb or reliquary was not to gaze: it was to touch, albeit indirectly.

Sumption cites an example that shows just how tangible this force was imagined to be. Gregory of Tours provided advice to any pilgrim who planned to visit the tomb of Saint Peter in Rome: "Should he wish to bring back a relic from the tomb, he carefully weighs a piece of cloth which he then hangs inside the tomb. Then he prays ardently and, if his faith is sufficient, the cloth, once removed from the tomb, will be found to be so full of divine grace that it will be much heavier than before."[38]

Given that *virtus* was considered to be a force much like gravity, one might infer that the larger the relic fragment, the greater the force it emitted. And in early Christianity this was indeed the predominant belief. Before the sixth century, a premium was placed on retaining the entire body of a saint and keeping it in a single shrine. To gain the intercession of the saint, pilgrimage to the shrine was required. Aron Gurevich explains that in the case of Martin of Tours, "one can speak of a 'force field' within the bounds of which the *virtus* of a saint was active. Martin's power to heal applied only so long as those who received it either came to Tours or remained there."[39]

Over time this belief was gradually replaced by the idea that any relic, no matter how minuscule, contained a force equal to the power of the whole.[40] The tiniest fragment of thread, the smallest sliver of bone, possessed the same *virtus* as an entire garment or the saint's entire skeleton. And with this shift in thinking came the introduction of another distinction, between primary and secondary relics. Primary relics were either corporeal remains of the saint or material objects with which the saint had had direct contact. Secondary relics, sometimes called *brandea*, consisted of any matter that might have had contact with a primary relic. Examples include particles of dust and morsels taken from the saint's tomb and water seeping from beneath it.[41] *Brandea* could generate yet other relics, as when dust particles from a saint's tomb or drops of blood from a martyred saint such as Thomas Becket were mixed with water: the water then became a relic with the same power to heal as the primary one.[42]

The reasons why these beliefs changed are not altogether clear (at least not to me). Nevertheless, the belief that a single part contained the same quantity of spiritual radioactivity as the whole made it possible to spread relics throughout the entire Christian world and thereby unify dispersed communities of worshippers, an objective that might otherwise have been very difficult to achieve.

The beliefs surrounding the force of *virtus* were elaborated in other ways. For example, it was believed that relics could be transported to different places without diminishing their potency. At the same time, a relic's power to heal depended on keeping it enclosed, no matter where it was. If it was exposed to the open air, its powers would dissipate. Thus, though bits and pieces of saints' relics could be found throughout the Christian world, they were always encased and displayed in tombs and boxes.

Medieval notions about saints represent an intriguing amalgam of powers and elements from the two realms, heaven and earth, where the saints were said to reside and have agency. Guided by a process that has been described by modern-day cognitive scientists as "conceptual blending," these elements were brought together to create a unique entity, one that made it possible for ordinary people to access heavenly powers in this world.[43]

Registering the Appeal

The complicated system of beliefs about saints gave rise to ritual practices for establishing a relationship with a divine advocate. These are seen most clearly in the rules and conventions governing pilgrimage.

Before departing on pilgrimage, and en route, a supplicant would be expected to confess his sins. He would then visit the saint's relics and present gifts, pray before them, and achieve close contact with them by wrapping his body around the reliquary that housed them, inserting afflicted body parts into special holes carved in the sides of the saint's tomb, or sleeping beside it. In prayers the supplicant would indicate the nature of the miracle sought and would remain at the pilgrimage site for days or even weeks. If the saint consented to intercede on his behalf, and if God acceded to the saint's request, a miracle would be granted.

THE ROLE OF HUMAN AGENCY
IN MIRACLES AND SAINTS

Little of the agency involved in miracles was assigned to ordinary people. The power to affect events in the world belonged almost entirely to God and the saints. Supplicants were humble, powerless beings subject to heavenly forces.

In one respect, however, this depiction is misleading: it overlooks the fact that human beings invented and composed the narrative in the first place. As one observer aptly puts it, "Sainthood is an eminently social phenomenon. Saints are made, not born. . . . [Saints] achieve positive recognition from their contemporaries."[44]

At first blush, this point may seem obvious. But on closer examination it appears that those who depict themselves in the narrative of sainthood as being without agency in fact had a prominent role in writing it. Moreover, those who represented themselves as being without a voice in the process largely determined who gained fame as a saint, and how, where, and when saints were venerated. Claims of miracles, after all, depend entirely on the words of ordinary people: it is they who act as publicists on behalf of some saints and not of others.

This insight first occurred to me while reading Patrick Geary's fascinating book *Furta Sacra*, which recounts the history of the robust and highly profitable trade in stolen relics during the medieval period. Stolen relics were in fact considered more valuable than those acquired by legitimate means. Because no self-respecting saint would ever allow her relics to be moved without her approval, a successful theft was taken as a sign that the saint had been unhappy with the previous earthly home of her relics and preferred the new location.[45] This belief was so powerful that monastic orders that had acquired relics in perfectly legitimate ways sometimes misrepresented them as stolen.[46] The community that owned an important relic was considered to be under the special protection of the saint in question, and thus anyone tempted to harm that community risked incurring the saint's wrath.[47] The extraordinary means the saint had chosen to reach this final resting place were thought to validate the community's rights to ownership and protection. In Gurevich's words, "The saint is the property of the inhabitants of the particular locality where his relics repose."[48]

One aspect of the practice of relic theft is puzzling. Why would saints be thought to connive at theft, even by their most devoted followers? If they really wanted their relics moved, why would they require human assistance? They were routinely credited with all sorts of other fantastic interventions in events: calming storms in midcycle, performing rescues at sea, ending epidemics and famines, repelling invasions, curing illness instantaneously, even reviving the dead. Though humans always depicted their role in such translations as passive, even accidental, in this one respect, saints were apparently without agency. For relics to move from one location to another, humans had to collect and transport them.

This puzzling inconsistency caused me to think further about human agency in the medieval cult of saints. When I began to look, human handprints appeared everywhere. I realized that far from being the passive bystanders they believed they were, humans were instead its principal authors.

The Hands of Humans in Reports about Miracles

It was human beings, not saints (or even God), who effectively dictated the precise *forms* that miracles took. They held ideas both about things saints could do and about things they could not do. We know that people accorded saints agency in curing fevers, leprosy, blindness, and deafness; providing relief from crippling conditions; and enabling recovery from accidents. Yet they apparently would have considered it strange to ask the saints to restore amputated limbs or lost teeth, to make old people young, to turn children into adults, or to enhance a supplicant's physical strength, height, beauty, or intelligence. Perhaps such prayers were offered but never recorded. It is far more likely, however, that humans had well-defined ideas about the limits of the saints' powers.

Similarly, the form that a miracle took was determined less by the saint than by the supplicant's request. That is, supplicants did not pray to the saint for a miracle and then leave it up to the saint to decide what sort of benefit might be in the recipient's best spiritual or personal interest. Instead they asked for quite specific things: restore my sight, heal my wounds, cure my leprosy, relieve my stomach pains, cause harm to my enemies. One might imagine that saints, through their special relationship with God, might have been attributed with the ability to facilitate a wide range of miraculous things, but would not do so unless asked. In modern terms, the nature of the miracles was driven by demand rather than supply.

Other evidence of human agency is apparent in the ways miracles were reported and judged. A determination of sainthood depended crucially on whether the candidate was considered instrumental in causing miracles to occur; indeed, a miracle cure was taken as proof positive of sanctity. But where did the evidence for miracle cures come from? In the overwhelming majority of cases, these accounts were supplied by ordinary people, who presented them to shrine keepers to record in their books. Whereas in the modern period claims of miracles have been subjected to investigation by experts in several fields, no such procedure existed in medieval times. The proof of miracles rested entirely on what ordinary people said. In this sense, the ontological existence of the saint hinged on the word of the supplicant.

Thus human beings were in a sense dictating what miracles they wanted done and then providing the evidence that they actually happened; the entire proof and justification of the wondrous powers of God and the saints rested with the human observer.

The Role of Humans in Making Saints

The role humans play in the institution of sainthood, both medieval and modern, goes beyond individuals' reporting miraculous events. After the earliest years of Christianity, whether an individual attained

sainthood typically depended on vigorous efforts by publicists and propagandists who wrote about the saint, recorded miracles attributed to
him, and spread the story of the saint's accomplishments far and wide.
Even if local inhabitants were aware of these achievements, without
such efforts, no deceased individual could become known as a saint.

Accounts of saints and their shrines commonly include some mention of these publicists.[49] For example, for a brief time during the thirteenth century, one of the most popular pilgrimage sites in England
was the tomb of the boy martyr William of Norwich. William had
three propagandists, the chief one being Thomas of Monmouth, a
monk affiliated with the church in which William was ultimately buried. Miracles attributed to Thomas Becket were recorded and publicly
proclaimed by two monks of Canterbury, Benedict and William. The
monks of Durham were responsible for publicizing miracles ascribed to
Godric of Finchale and to Cuthbert. The saint of Hereford Cathedral,
the thirteenth-century bishop Thomas of Cantilupe, had as his advocate
his successor as bishop, Richard Swinfield. Swithin's miracles were publicized by the entire body of monks of Winchester Cathedral. Edmund
of Abingdon's miracles were narrated by the Cistercian monks of Pontigny, where he had died. Hugh of Lincoln gained renown through the
efforts of his chaplain, Adam the Monk, who issued the *Magna Vita* of
1212. Wulfstan of Worcester was memorialized in the writings of William of Malmesbury. The list goes on.[50]

Thomas of Monmouth's efforts to commemorate William of Norwich
illustrate the lengths to which publicists sometimes went. William came
from a small village nearby and at an early age was apprenticed to a leather
worker in the city of Norwich. In 1144 he went missing, and his body
eventually turned up in a wooded area on the edge of the city.[51] His death
attracted little attention, and he was buried unceremoniously in a grave
near the spot where his body was found. But when a rumor spread that
William had been the victim of a ritual murder by the Jews of Norwich,
interest in him began to grow. His remains were moved to the cathedral
cemetery, and before long reports began to emerge of miracles associated

with visits to his tomb. In 1150 Thomas of Monmouth became a monk at Norwich Cathedral and, for reasons no one fully understands, proclaimed himself William's chief propagandist. He sought out witnesses to miracles, recorded their stories, and publicized them. He even tried to precipitate miracles by bringing people to the tomb to venerate William, in one case offering tomb dust mixed in water as a cure for someone who was ill. He kept at this task until he died in 1170.

In the later Middle Ages, the role of human agency in naming saints began to change. After the second decade of the thirteenth century, saints owed their status almost entirely to propagandists, because Pope Innocent III's proclamation of 1215 gave the Roman Curia exclusive authority to canonize. Thereafter canonization required increasingly elaborate, time-consuming, and costly procedures, including taking testimony from numerous witnesses and filing formal petitions to the curia and the College of Cardinals before seeking the approval of the pope.[52] As the Church tightened its control over the process of canonization, the number of new saints dropped dramatically: according to one study, between 1198 and 1432, the rate of canonization dropped from one new saint every 3.1 years to one every 13.5 years.[53] The historian Ben Nilson explains that many canonization attempts failed for lack of money and influence, even though the candidate saints had thriving cults of followers.[54]

This is a point worth our pausing to think about. If, as the commonly accepted narrative implies, saints are identified by God, then why would numbers drop over time? Had God simply turned off the supply of sanctity for a time, had the supply of virtuous people begun to dry up, or did the stream slow because of the actions of humans? (To maintain some perspective on this question, we should remember that during the twenty-six-year rule of Pope John Paul II [1978–2004], some 1,339 persons were beatified [the first step toward canonization], and 483 were canonized: more saints were proclaimed in this period than by all popes from the late Middle Ages until the 1970s.)[55]

The role of saints' propagandists was constrained by the limited means for spreading the word. The emergence of the mass media changed the task entirely. The shrine at Lourdes in the French Pyrenees was established following an apparition of the Virgin reported by a local peasant girl, Bernadette Soubirous, in 1858. At the time, Lourdes was a small, obscure village, and at first only a few locals made it a site of pilgrimage. In 1866, the Missionaries of Notre Dame de Garaison took over its administration and began to publicize it aggressively in the French Catholic press.[56] Ruth Harris explains how vigorously they pursued their mission: "In Lourdes between 1867 and 1877, 'every Sunday, at the two o'clock service, the request for prayers that [the Garaison Fathers] had received and the cases of divine grace were read out.' Scores of narratives . . . were sent to the fathers, either by the *miraculés* themselves or by their priests and other interested lay people. . . . Others were printed in the *Annales de Notre-Dame de Lourdes*, which recounted at least a dozen and sometimes as many as forty cures per year between 1873 and 1883."[57]

Lourdes was promoted through newspapers, guidebooks, and other publications. The Internet has introduced an entirely new medium for promoting saints. Searching for Padre Pio, an Italian monk who lived from 1887 to 1968 and was proclaimed a saint in 2002, produces some 2,740,000 Google listings. The shrine in Medjugorje in Bosnia yields 1,220,000 listings. This shrine became famous because of a Marian apparition experienced by six young people in June 1981. The anthropologist Paolo Apolito, who has studied it, concludes: "With Medjugorje, we are dealing with one of the most powerful publicity campaigns ever conducted around a religious phenomenon." The same source provides a fascinating account of the use of the web for promoting information about contemporary Marian apparitions.[58]

Bargaining and Bickering with Saints

Further evidence of the role of conscious human agency in sainthood is supplied by the phenomenon of supplicants bargaining with saints. In many cases, particularly in the later Middle Ages, supplicants tried to strike deals with the saints they venerated. They would pray to saints not at their shrines but at local parish churches. In their prayers, they offered to undertake a pilgrimage to the saint's shrine and leave gifts provided that the saint first produced a miracle. Conversely, they might threaten to abandon their veneration of one saint in favor of another unless the desired miracle was forthcoming.

Bargaining also took other forms. Citing a source from the ninth-century life of Bishop Rigobert of Reims, Gurevich recounts the story of a woman suffering from a fever who attempted to put the saints to a test. She asked three different saints for help and then lit three candles of equal length, one for each of them, intending to gauge the comparative power of the saints by seeing how long the candles burned. The candle of one of the saints burned longer than the others, and so the woman prayed to him, presented him with gifts, and received the desired result.[59]

Interestingly, these practices are not recorded from the early centuries of Christianity, perhaps because the list of saints was then comparatively small and their credentials were considered beyond dispute. By the late Middle Ages, however, claims to sainthood depended almost entirely on the testimony of ordinary persons, and thus they were perceived to have sufficient leverage to bargain with the saints.

The passive and powerless role traditionally assigned to supplicants is thus somewhat misleading. When we examine how rituals were enacted in practice, and the actions of those who attempted to establish and retain beneficial relationships with saints, we find evidence of a considerable degree of conscious agency by humans. The institution of sainthood was a human creation designed to fulfill a vital social function.

CHAPTER THREE

Apparitions

Although people may fervently believe in the idea of divine protection for the living, beliefs by themselves don't suffice. Also seemingly needed is concrete, tangible evidence of a divine presence in the human midst. The impression that heaven is present in some form on earth may be created and sustained in any number of ways: with impressive tombs and ornately decorated reliquaries where music, art, and incense foster an aura of the saints' presence; through publicizing of miracles that reportedly take place in connection with venerating saints; and as apparitions, in which figures such as Christ, the Virgin Mary, or an important saint appear in visions.

The study of saints, their relics, and the miracles ascribed to them can tell us much about the role ordinary humans play in creating and sustaining the impression of a divine presence on earth. Yet firsthand accounts have limited value. By definition, the divine status of great saints is seen by worshippers as beyond dispute. True believers accept uncritically the dramatic events ascribed to saints. Consequently, stories about the cult of saints and the miracles they perform tend to conceal the role of humans in creating and sustaining the impression of a heavenly presence.

Reports about apparitions, by contrast, are often met with skepticism, and ridicule, if not outright disbelief. Written records tell us how

49

these doubts have been addressed and skeptics eventually won over. Reports of apparitions record who experienced them, when and where they occurred, the heavenly figure or figures that appeared to the visionaries, what form the apparition took, how news of it was received by bystanders, how visionaries' initial reports were transformed from often vague stories to coherent accounts, the figure's reasons for appearing, and the message he or she wished to transmit to the visionary's community and beyond. These accounts also show how visionaries' standing in the community changes when reports begin to be accepted as true. They are treated as heroes, quasi-saints, local ambassadors to heaven. And their communities are transformed as well. Such visions thus produce a script for a rich, intricate drama that underscores the impression that heaven has appeared on earth.

WHEN SAINTS APPEAR

The early history of Christianity is replete with instances of religious hermits, ascetics, and others reporting visions of Christ or a major saint suddenly appearing to them, often while they were alone in some remote place. Similar visions have occurred closer to the modern age to less exceptional human beings. Famous examples include the repeated apparition of the Virgin Mary to two shepherd children at La Salette, a remote village high in the French Alps near Grenoble, in 1846; the apparition of the Virgin at Lourdes in 1858 to the twelve-year-old Bernadette Soubirous; and the Virgin's apparition in 1917 at Fátima, a village in Portugal, to three young children.[1]

Appearances by the Virgin were reported throughout the twentieth century and continue today. For example, she allegedly appeared to an adult woman, Rosa Quattrini, in the southern Italian village of San Damiano in 1964 (though this account has been much disputed); to four young girls in the Spanish village of San Sebastián de Garabandal in 1961; and to six young children in the Bosnian village of Medjugorje beginning in 1981 and continuing for some time.[2] According to one source, from 1945 to 1999, there were 692 such events reported around the world, in Slovakia, Hungary, Bosnia, Portugal, Spain, Belgium, Malta, Italy, Holland, Germany, France, the United Kingdom, Egypt, Rwanda, Brazil, Venezuela, Argentina, Mexico, Puerto Rico, India, China, Japan, the Philippines, Canada, and, in the United States, in California, Indiana, New York, Missouri, Florida, New Mexico, Minnesota, Ohio, and Illinois.[3]

Most modern visionary experiences are described in some form of written account, such as a newspaper story, an autobiography, or an article in a religious journal. Though written reports of apparitions from the medieval period also survive, for our purposes they are of limited value because they tend to be highly truncated, unelaborated claims by individuals in remote settings and unsupported by evidence from others. Moreover, they generally lack any context that might yield clues about why the apparitions occurred when and to whom they did. Because accounts of contemporary apparitions are far more complete, I rely on them here to describe the kind of social and cultural work that apparitions perform.

Lourdes: The Prototype

The appearance in 1858 of the Virgin to Bernadette Soubirous at Lourdes is paradigmatic of most other modern-day Marian apparitions and serves as a useful introduction to the topic. Bernadette claimed that the Virgin appeared to her eighteen times near Lourdes between February and July. All the visions happened at the same location, in the hollow of a rock in a grotto, and each involved the appearance of a young woman whom Bernadette initially described as *aqueró*, translated roughly as "that one."[4] Though she was sometimes accompanied by others while experiencing these apparitions, only Bernadette was able to see the visions she described; this is a feature characteristic of apparition stories.

On one of these occasions, the vision instructed Bernadette to uncover a previously unknown spring at the site of the grotto. One

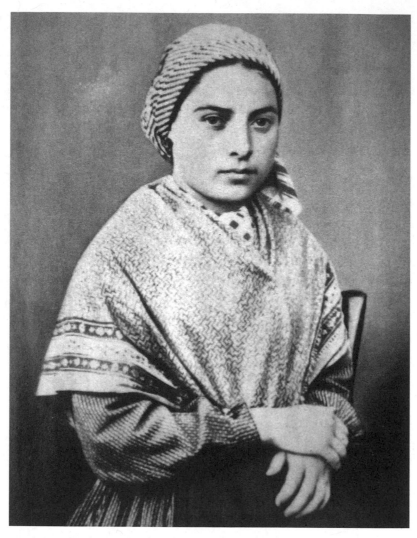

Figure 3.   Bernadette Soubirous, the visionary of Lourdes. Wikimedia
Commons.

authoritative source, however, points out that some locals—including a pig herder, a sawyer, several fishermen, and a number of farmers—claimed to have known of a spring at the site well before Bernadette's visions.[5] On another occasion the image instructed her to tell the local priest that the Virgin wished to have a chapel built on the spot and for processions to be made to it. At first the local clergy dismissed her claims as fantastic, but in time they came to accept them as true—in part, perhaps, because the grotto was fast becoming a major attraction to pilgrims not only from the immediate area but, thanks to newspaper coverage, from the whole of France. Four years after Bernadette's first apparition, in 1862, the local bishop proclaimed that her reports were valid and ordered a basilica to be built on the site. A decade later, the annual pilgrimages to Lourdes were instituted, drawing the faithful from all over France and elsewhere in Europe.

Except for brief periods during the two world wars, pilgrimages to Lourdes have continued to the present day. By the end of 1908, which marked the fiftieth anniversary of the apparitions, some 5,297 pilgrimage groups had officially registered with the shrine keepers, together bringing an estimated 4.9 million pilgrims. These included some who were seriously ill and in search of cures, and others (probably the majority) who accompanied them on their journey. The visitors also included individual pilgrims, who perhaps outnumbered those who came in groups, and tourists simply interested in visiting a place of spiritual renown. Lourdes has become one of the most famous and frequently visited healing shrines of the modern age.

Lourdes did not begin as a healing shrine: it was simply a place where an apparition had occurred. According to Ruth Harris, "There was nothing in the Virgin's message suggesting such a possibility [of miracle cures]—the injunction to build a chapel, come in processions, pray for sinners and bathe and drink at the grotto held no promise of miracles."[6] Indeed, in 1858, sensing a business opportunity arising from the site's recent fame, the local mayor briefly toyed with the idea of converting the spring into a secular health spa of a type common elsewhere in the

Pyrenees. He even commissioned a hydrologist to analyze the waters of the grotto, which (unhappily for him) indicated that they contained no unusual mineral qualities.[7]

Nevertheless, local inhabitants who flocked to the grotto after Bernadette's visions to bathe in its water reported the first cures associated with Lourdes, and the local bishop came to accept the apparitions as real. Within ten years Lourdes had begun to gain renown as a healing shrine. A Paris-based religious order, the Augustinian Fathers of the Assumption, was assigned responsibility for managing the shrine. With the help of the expanding railway network and the Catholic popular press, the Assumptionist Fathers transformed Lourdes into a site of mass pilgrimage.[8] By the early 1900s, close to half a million pilgrims, mainly women from rural France, came to Lourdes on church-sponsored national pilgrimages each year. Thus, within fifty years of Bernadette's experiences, the previously unknown village of Lourdes had been transformed into one of the most famous pilgrimage sites in the Christian world.[9]

THE SOCIOLOGY OF APPARITIONS

Because of events reported from Lourdes, La Salette, Fátima, and other modern apparitional sites, people today generally associate such visions with appearances of the Virgin. But this has not always been the case. Reports of apparitions before the eleventh century were almost always of Christ or one of the apostles, or sometimes a martyr or confessor. Only in the eleventh and twelfth centuries did the Virgin begin to appear to people.[10] Sightings were regularly reported until the sixteenth century. After that, she seems to have disappeared from view until the middle of the nineteenth century. This pattern bears a striking relationship to important developments in Western Christianity, such as the emergence and flourishing of the cult of the Virgin shortly before the first millennium, the Protestant Reformation of the sixteenth century, and the reemergence of Catholic fundamentalism in the nineteenth century in reaction to the Enlightenment.[11] Though we might be tempted to conclude that this pattern of reported appearances is due to shifts in religious thinking and practice, true believers are apt to believe that she was appearing to people all the while but that visionaries were reluctant to speak out about their experiences during periods of religious oppression.

Modern-day accounts of apparitions of the Virgin raise questions about the part played by humans in constructing them, an instance of what modern-day sociologists and anthropologists commonly describe as "the social construction of reality."[12] Signs of human agency abound in accounts of Marian apparitions. In one famous case in sixteenth-century Spain, apparitions, visions, and miracles occurred in connection with what later turned out to be false documents. At the end of the sixteenth century, a set of documents was reportedly found recounting the alleged discovery by a professor at the nearby University of Baezby that two fourth-century Christian martyrs had been tortured and killed by a Roman governor in A.D. 308 at a castle in Arjona for refusing to renounce their faith. Over the next several decades, the bogus revelation that the two martyrs had once lived in the village gave rise to a series of apparitions and reports of other supernatural events. Certain that the martyrs were buried near the base of the castle wall, local authorities began excavations that turned up human bones, ashes, and artifacts that were said to be instruments of torture. As more and more relics were uncovered, pilgrims were drawn to the site, and reports of miracle cures began to circulate. Before long, Arjona became a place of pilgrimage and gained renown as a healing shrine. At the very end of the seventeenth century, the chronicles recounting the legend were exposed as forgeries, and with this revelation pilgrimages to the site died out.[13]

To explore the role of human agency in apparitions of the Virgin and other saints, we need to understand a difference between the sites of apparitions and the sites of the tombs of great saints. The tombs that house the bodies or relics of famous saints are usually housed in great churches in or near large urban areas: for example, the burial place of Saint James at Compostela, or the shrine of Thomas Becket at Canterbury Cathedral. For local residents and those with the wherewithal to undertake pilgrimages, these are convenient sites for seeking miracle cures, gaining divine protection, or fulfilling spiritual needs. But what of poorer people and those who reside in remote villages? Their thirst for a saint's benevolent protection is every bit as great as that of others, but their poverty and isolation mean that other ways must be found (some believe invented) for achieving it. An apparition involving the dramatic appearance of the Virgin or another famous heavenly figure is one such mechanism.

William Christian's study of apparitions of the late medieval and early Renaissance periods in Spain succinctly explains the dynamics of this process. Christian explains that during medieval and preindustrial times in rural Spain, village life was fraught with natural and man-made sources of danger: epidemics, earthquakes, droughts, floods, accidents and fires, raids by marauders. And, as in most medieval communities, civic and social institutions offered little protection against these myriad sources of harm. For help, people turned to heaven.

Christian portrays the medieval God as a terrifying, all-powerful, vengeful figure. Sickness, famine, earthquakes, and pestilence were all interpreted as God's punishments for sins. This conception of an angry God enables us to make sense of bizarre-seeming features of common religious practices. Penitential processions by representatives of the entire community were common, most often led by flagellants. These individuals believed that by punishing themselves—whipping their own bodies, slashing their skin, tearing their flesh, wearing crowns of thorns, crawling on their hands and knees, even starving themselves—they might persuade God that it would be unnecessary for him to administer further punishment.[14]

But flagellation and other penitential rituals could take a community only so far. Whatever else they might accomplish, such acts offered no assurance that beings in heaven were paying the slightest attention. And yet, as Christian reminds us, "for communities involved in a relentless series of epidemics and crop failures, this was a matter of life and death."[15] It is at the nexus of these concerns that we begin to glimpse the important social and cultural work that apparitions perform.

Where Apparitions Take Place

Apparitions most often occur in communities that feel they lack ready access to heavenly protection. Under these circumstances, people begin to reach out to saints: apparitions confirm that these appeals have not been in vain, that contact has indeed been made. In Christian's words, through apparitions, heavenly beings are "communicating their availability and benevolent interest."[16] Saints who appear in visions are understood to be offering their services to the community.

Most recorded apparitions have occurred in remote settings, mainly rural villages. Even today, the population of La Salette, where the Virgin reportedly appeared in 1846, is no more than two hundred people. At the time of Bernadette's vision of the Virgin in 1858, Lourdes had a population of only four thousand, and at the time of the apparition at Fátima in 1917, the community was described as little more than a small village. San Sebastián de Garabandal, a rural village in northern Spain where the Virgin first reportedly appeared in 1961, has a population of three hundred. Oliveto Citra, near Salerno, where the Virgin appeared in 1985, has a current population of about four thousand people,[17] and Medjugorje, where the Virgin began appearing in 1981, then had a population of about the same size.

Travel brochures and Internet sites advertising places where Marian apparitions have reportedly occurred tend to describe the Virgin's dramatic appearance in similar ways. But closer examination of the details surrounding these events paints a picture that is more complicated, ambiguous, and interesting.

Visionaries Who See Saints

All alleged modern-day visionaries were young children at the time of the apparitions, and generally they are reported as not at first identifying the apparition as the Virgin. Either they described a unique but vaguely defined visual experience or, if they described a human figure, they could not identify it. For example, the visionaries at La Salette told people that they had seen a bright light with an oval face, hands, arms, and elbows, but not the rest of the figure. The children referred to the figure not as the Virgin, but only as "a beautiful lady." Bernadette referred to the figure in her famous apparition at Lourdes as "that one." At Fátima, the children said that they had seen a figure of some sort, but one that appeared to them to be like "a statue made of snow . . . rendered almost transparent by the rays of the sun." When one of these visionaries, Lúcia, told her mother about it, she said that it looked like a person wrapped in a sheet and that she could not make out any eyes or hands. Initially she referred to the apparitional figure as "a pretty little woman." The youthful visionaries associated with other sites of Marian apparitions use similar phrases, referring to bright images, a "beautiful lady," or simply "strange lights," but never "the Virgin."[18]

How, then, and by whom, were these visual experiences labeled as apparitions of the Virgin? In most cases it was adults in the community who made the identification, often the visionaries' mothers, close relatives, neighbors, or sometimes journalists. According to Sandra Zimdars-Swartz, the typical pattern is for children to report strange sightings and for adults to tell them what they have seen. As word of the vision spreads, the identity of the apparition becomes established as fact. The children themselves also now retrospectively "realize" the true identity of the figure in their visions.[19] And, of course, once the children proclaim that it is the Virgin who has appeared, they are on the way to becoming sacred celebrities.

Not all those to whom the Virgin has appeared were children at the time. The visionaries studied by William Christian in Spain include farmers, herders, and hunters, and others who work alone and in remote settings. He also reports cases of Marian appearances experienced by milkmen, sailors, fishermen, domestic servants, factory workers, housewives, and local mystics.[20]

All these people share one characteristic: they were living on the margins of their small communities.[21] One prominent member of the

Lourdes community described the Soubirous family as "miserable people," saying that "their language, especially their habits and their reputation" were such as to "destroy the charm [of the apparition story], inspiring not only doubt but disgust."[22]

The reason why visions are typically ascribed to the powerless and marginalized has invited intense speculation. One common hypothesis is that the visionaries' lowly status leaves them immune from the suspicion of having some personal or political agenda to advance. The motives of a bishop, a parish priest, a local merchant, or a public official reporting an apparition might well be suspect. The fact that the source of the story is someone who symbolizes innocence and humility lends credence to the message.[23]

The cases of child visionaries are especially intriguing. The visionaries of La Salette were a girl, age fourteen, and a boy, age eleven. The visionary of Lourdes, Bernadette Soubirous, was twelve years old when she reported her encounter with the figure she initially identified alternatively either as *aqueró* or "jeune fille."[24] The oldest of the three visionaries at Fátima was ten years of age. At San Sebastián, the four girls associated with the apparition of the Virgin were twelve, eleven, and younger, and all six of the visionaries at Medjugorje were children. Reports invariably suggest that their backgrounds may have been related to the visions. According to her autobiography, the young shepherdess who was one of the two visionaries at La Salette had a very difficult childhood. She was rejected by her mother, who locked her out of house for days at a time and eventually told the child that she was no longer considered a member of the family. Her employer characterized her as "extremely lazy, disobedient and sullen," someone who refused to respond when spoken to and who often hid in the fields near her home all night. The other La Salette visionary, a twelve-year-old shepherd boy, is also described as having had an unhappy childhood. His mother died when he was eighteen months old; his father remarried shortly thereafter, and he was abused by his stepmother, who described him as reckless and without foresight.[25] Bernadette Soubirous of Lourdes endured a similarly difficult childhood. Because her father was a drunk-ard who could not hold a regular job, her family was forced to live with relatives in conditions of dire poverty. Shortly before the age of twelve, she was hired out as a shepherdess to spare her family the expense of feeding her. She was a sickly child, suffering from chronic asthma and disorders associated with malnutrition.[26]

The chief visionary of Fátima was Lúcia dos Santos. The story of her early childhood adds an additional element of intrigue. In her memoirs, it begins cheerfully: she describes herself as gifted with talents that were apparent from the earliest age. One of these was an ability to entertain people of all ages, and another was an ability to get people to do what she wanted them to do. She recounts the pleasure she gained from entertain-ing people at local festivals and fairs by singing and dancing for them and telling stories. The other two visionaries of Fátima were her younger cousins: both became very attached to Lúcia, who regaled them with sto-ries, particularly fairy tales. Lúcia's mother considered her to be a special child and repeatedly told her to ask God to make her a saint. Then, at age seven, her status in the family changed abruptly. She was suddenly treated as being no different from her brothers and sister; she was summarily turned out and put in charge of herding the family's small flock of sheep.[27]

It is, of course, impossible to judge whether these childhood circum-stances were exceptional. It strikes me as plausible, however, that the rejection, cruelty, and hardships the children suffered played some role in the timing and content of the apparitions they experienced. If nothing else, these events would have made them highly receptive to participa-tion in a social drama that offered them the possibility of an escape from their plight. All of them had recently completed the catechism and taken first communion when they experienced their visions. Thus their newly acquired knowledge of their religion, coupled with a strong desire to escape their circumstances, might have rendered them highly receptive to the idea of declaring themselves the instruments of the Virgin.

In every case, only the children claimed to see the Virgin. Other peo-ple later accompanied them to the site where the Virgin had appeared but never saw her for themselves. Descriptions of such visits refer to crowds of curious onlookers demanding to know what the Virgin was telling the visionaries and pleading with them to appeal on the witnesses' behalf for favors and miracles.[28] In one instance at Melleray in the Republic of Ireland in 1985, two young boys claimed that the Virgin had appeared to them and told them that they were to receive messages from her on each of the next four nights. On the second day, friends and neighbors began to gather where the first apparition had taken place, near a Cistercian monastery at a grotto not unlike the one at Lourdes. By the end of the week, the crowds had grown to the thousands, and the demands for information from witnesses became so insistent that a public-address system was set up to enable the boys to repeat what the Virgin was saying to them.[29]

Imaginary Companions and Secrets

The phenomenon of children who report having had conversations with the Virgin may strike us as strange, but similar events are not unusual. One study estimates that 65 percent of all children talk to, play with, confide in, give gifts to, and receive instructions from imaginary companions.[30]

Studies of such imaginary friendships almost always include some mention of secrets. Although children seem to have no reluctance to tell others about an imaginary companion, they almost always allude to secrets that are shared strictly between the child and the imaginary friend. Secrets are also a striking feature of the conversations reported by child visionaries with the Virgin. Whether they encounter her on their own or in a group, these children claim that the Virgin has told them things they are to tell no one else.

Secrets are a common feature of social relationships. The sociologist Georg Simmel refers to them as " inner property," a resource children and adults use in an attempt to exercise power and influence over others.[31] The anthropologist Lorel Lindstrom points out that someone privy to a secret, by definition, knows something others do not know.

By constructing hidden worlds filled with messages shared only between imaginary confidantes, the holders of secrets employ a resource that helps them resist and reject supervision from above.[32]

Secrets entail two kinds of knowledge: the fact that a secret exists, and the fact that only certain people know what it is. The "paradox of secrecy" is that for a secret to have an effect on others, the fact of its existence must be revealed while the contents remain undisclosed.[33] The telling and keeping of secrets is common among young children, typically viewed as a mechanism not only for wresting from adults control over certain aspects of their lives but also for solidifying relationships between friends by excluding others.[34]

The anthropologist Tanya Luhrmann asserts that secrets are all about control. "By keeping something hidden from other people, secrecy elevates the value of the thing concealed. That which is kept hidden grows desirable and seems more powerful." Secrets also make it possible for children to experience independence: "Learning that it is possible to keep a secret teaches a child that he is an independent self who has some control over his world."[35]

The secrets associated with Marian apparitions bear the hallmarks of this familiar childhood practice. Yet Marian apparitions entail no ordinary secrets: messages from the Virgin might indicate her willingness to protect people from harm or reveal what they must do to avert the wrath of God.

At Medjugorje in 1981, the six young visionaries claimed that the Virgin had shared secrets with them and would continue to do so for some time to come. They explained that the secrets were of three types: personal secrets that concerned only the seers and would not be revealed publicly; matters of public interest but not of apparent great importance; and crucial secrets that allegedly pertained to the Roman Catholic Church and the whole world. The seers also told people that Mary had promised to confide ten secrets to each of them, after which she would then appear to that seer infrequently.[36] One of the seers, Ivan Dragicevic, still claims to experience apparitions almost thirty years later. He now spends half of each year in the United States giving talks to interested audiences and describing his continuing visions.[37]

In all cases, child visionaries seem to have taken action to disseminate the news that they were privy to divine secrets, along with affirming their unwillingness to reveal the secrets. Inevitably, adults have tried to get the children to tell, sometimes engaging in almost inquisitorial techniques: local priests and bishops have cajoled them, isolated them, and even threatened them with eternal damnation. The children's resolute refusal to give up the secrets has generally only added credence to their claims.[38]

Crowds

A visionary's report that the Virgin has promised to return at a specified time and place naturally causes great local excitement. These prognostications have resulted in huge crowds of followers accompanying the seer to the appointed site. At Lourdes, within days of Bernadette's announcement that her initial apparition had been followed by others, crowds numbering in the thousands began to accompany her to the grotto where she first saw the Virgin. At Fátima, six months after the two children had reported their visions of the Virgin, crowds estimated at seventy thousand began to appear. Similarly huge crowds formed at San Sebastián.[39]

As with many secrets and tall tales, these revelations gained a momentum of their own. As the child visionaries told their stories, the stakes mounted, and they were under great pressure to deliver accounts of further apparitions. The apparitions had been transformed in their minds, and the minds of others, from amorphous bright lights and unidentifiable figures to confirmed sightings of the Virgin. This transformation required the convincing of skeptical adults, who thereby also acquired a stake in confirming and perpetuating the accounts. At La Salette, at first no one put any stock at all in the children's story. At Lourdes, some looked upon Bernadette as having been deceived by the devil. The seers at San Sebastián were taunted by other children in the village and

questioned harshly by the local priest about what they said they had
seen; a close relative of one of them called her account "absolute folly."
Anecdotes like these help us understand the magnitude of the personal
stakes involved for the visionaries.[40] Indeed, one shudders to imagine
what might have happened to the children if they had announced that
the Virgin had failed to reappear as promised at a specified time and
place. These pressures, and the fact that no one else was able to see the
Virgin, lend credence to the view that childhood imagination has played
a major role in shaping such events.

The Marian visions display another common characteristic of collective behavior: the tendency for one highly publicized instance to give
rise to a rash of similar events. Paolo Apolito explains: "Every case of
an apparition that has attained a certain level of renown has soon produced a sort of visionary 'epidemic' in the surrounding territory. It happened in the past at Lourdes, it happened at Fátima, and it happened
in Belgium following the apparitions of Beauring and Nabbeux, in the
years 1932 and 1933, which in the year 1933 alone produced twelve
phenomena of imitative visions." In his study of Oliveto Citra, the small
town near Salerno where the Virgin appeared, Apolito identifies imitative events in nine other nearby towns.[41]

Establishing the Sacredness of the Apparitional Site

The standard accounts of apparition have an additional feature that powerfully reinforces the gradually emerging story: the stubborn refusal of
the Virgin to allow the establishment of a pilgrimage site anywhere but
at the location of the apparition. Some apparitions involve the discovery
of statues or other material proofs of the visit. Where these appear, the
saint is often portrayed as refusing to allow the objects to be moved. William Christian reports a pattern among the reports of nearly one hundred apparitions involving the discovery of statues and other religious
icons: when such artifacts were moved, say, to the local parish church,
they were somehow miraculously returned to their original location. For

example, a shepherd finding a statue in a field or glen might place it in his pouch or knapsack and bring it to the parish priest. The priest might accept it and lock it in a chest in the village church; the next day, the image might be found missing and discovered to have returned to its original site in the countryside.[42] If villagers tried to build a shrine to house the object away from the site where it was found, the construction materials might mysteriously vanish overnight and reappear at the site where the apparition occurred. Such myths underscore the impression that the saint is proclaiming to the world that the apparitional site is the only place where his or her presence and protection can be experienced.[43]

This pattern is in marked contrast to the beliefs and practices surrounding the tombs of great saints. Though it was not initially the case, by the tenth century, tombs and the reliquaries that housed saints' bones and other body parts were considered to be fully transportable. Bones and detritus connected to great saints were moved from one location to another with considerable dispatch. Cathedrals, monastic churches, and other great churches could give away parts of relics. (Reading Abbey in England was once famous for possessing a finger of Saint James, whose other remains were entombed at Compostela.) In fact, there is an entire ceremonial ritual, known as a translation, for moving the tomb or relics of a great saint, with the saint's aura of sacredness going with it. But it seems that sites of apparitions are not, as it were, geographically fungible, contributing to the impression that ordinary people living in these otherwise anonymous settlements are under the special protection of the saint that appears among them.

The Celebrity of the Visionaries

When visionaries manage to attract believers, other consequences follow. Celebrity quickly supplants marginality and anonymity. To quote Christian's apt phrase, they are granted "ambassadorship to heaven," the status of a "chosen person." Children become quasi-saints who can mediate with the Virgin for special graces and favors for the faithful.[44]

In medieval times (and still today), reports of miracles helped legitimize of claims about sacred and holy spaces: they were taken as proof that a holy figure was in fact present at the site. Such miracles would not have been difficult to arrange, as Christian explains: "In every community, at any time, people have a number of everyday minor ailments, and some people suffer chronic infirmities. The quick curing of local people typically provided the initial impetus for the formation of a regional curing center."[45] The kinds of disorders for which miracle cures were claimed included "dolor de castado" (flank pain), rabies, hernia, eye disorders, ear infections, toothaches, a weak heart, seizures, sciatica, blindness, and, for women, a dangerous pregnancy.

The attractiveness of appealing to saints for cures was heightened by the starkness of the alternatives that were available to ordinary rural people. Where medical care was available at all, it consisted of such unpleasant and costly procedures as cauterization, bleeding, and hot poultices. "With this kind of competition," Christian writes, "the shrine at Cubas and others in early modern Spain flourished. At these shrines the fee was reasonable, it could be paid in kind, it was payable only if the cure was successful, and it was generally set by the patient."[46]

CONCLUSION

The work of contemporary scholars shows that apparitions—why, when, and how they appear, who reports them, and what happens in a community when people accept these reports as true—are more complicated and interesting phenomena than many accounts from the medieval period might lead us to believe. Such events are intimately connected with community life. Apparitions are mechanisms by which the imagined powers of heaven can be introduced into a community, no matter how anonymous and inconsequential it may be, and make their presence perceptible to the living.

CHAPTER FOUR

Pilgrimage and Shrines

I have explained why people turned to saints in search of cures for illnesses, and how they were expected to comport themselves in appealing for relief. I now take up another aspect of practices associated with
venerating saints: the custom of going on pilgrimage. This chapter
explains why people chose to go on pilgrimage and what such journeys
entailed.

Pilgrimage is hardly unique to Christianity. Other scholars—including students of religion, history, archaeology, and spirituality—have
written about it far more incisively that I could ever hope to do. By and
large, however, they are mainly concerned with the spiritual quest. My
own interest in the topic of pilgrimage is narrower. Though, of neces-
sity, it includes aspects of spiritual quests, I focus primarily on the beliefs
and practices associated with appealing to saints for relief from illness.

WHO WENT ON PILGRIMAGE?

According to Diana Webb, people of all classes participated in pilgrimage. Even the poorest made such journeys, often living off the charity
of monks and priests at churches along the way; some became quasi-
vagrants who took to the road and never left it. On long journeys, most

of the pilgrims were men. Women were more likely to engage in pilgrimages to local shrines.[1]

There were several reasons for this difference. One has to do with the role women played in looking after the home and the family. The dangers associated with long-distance travel raised concerns about sexual assault and violence. And finally, there was the practical objection that it was usually women who were trampled underfoot in the rush to venerate the relics of the Church.[2]

People joined pilgrimage for all sorts of reasons, illness being only one of them.[3] Most, including the sick, took to the road as a way of expressing devotion to their faith.[4] Some went involuntarily, having been ordered to make a pilgrimage by their bishop as a penance for their sins.[5] And, as one authority observes of pilgrimage: "At its center there remains the ancient draw of the supernatural and the miraculous, the desire to go, to sacrifice, to consult the oracle, to be a spectator at the common sanctuaries, to touch and experience, as part of a collective, the presence of the Divine in the places touched by the physical remains of particular persons who had enjoyed a particular intimacy with God as humans."[6] For some, of course, a pilgrimage was simply an excuse to travel.[7] It was one of the few accepted reasons for leaving one's work and responsibilities. Also, because monks at the pilgrimage churches along the route were expected to feed those who could not provide for themselves, such journeys offered the prospect of a partially subsidized vacation! Indeed, as traveling became easier and cheaper, tourism, thinly disguised as pilgrimage, became extremely popular.[8]

The Church offered incentives for pilgrimage. Indulgences (promises of a shortened sentence in purgatory) were commonly used to promote pilgrimages, particularly on major feast days and other notable anniversaries, and churches routinely petitioned their bishops to be allowed to grant up to forty days' worth of indulgence to enhance their appeal. Such tactics were often used to promote visits to newly established shrines.[9] One source describes how the bishop of Salisbury granted an indulgence of twenty days for any parishioner from his diocese who visited Thomas of Cantilupe's tomb at Hereford and contributed to the building fund, and another reports that in 1472–73, Pope Sixtus IV granted twelve years' indulgence to those who visited Salisbury Cathedral to celebrate the translation of Saint Osmund and paid a tax.[10]

CROWDS AT HEALING SHRINES

Given the many reasons why people might decide to join a pilgrimage, we should not be surprised that the more famous pilgrimage shrines attracted large crowds of worshippers. The various sites varied widely in popularity. Using a crude metric devised by the historian Ben Nilson to estimate crowd size at medieval healing shrines, based on an average gift of one penny per pilgrim, I calculate, for example, that at Etheldreda's shrine at the comparatively remote site of Ely in the years 1291–1360, visitors averaged 21 a day, or 7,680 a year. At Saint Edmund's shrine at Bury at the height of its popularity, the pilgrims' gifts, amounting to £120 a year, suggest annual visitors in the range of 28,800 people. At the shrine at Walsingham in Norfolk, which housed a relic containing a vial of the Virgin Mary's milk, the £260 in gifts pilgrims left in 1534 would imply 62,000 visits that year, an average of about 1,200 per week.[11]

At Becket's shrine at Canterbury, as I explained in my prologue, the crowds could be massive. Between 1198 and 1207, the average income from offerings was £309 per year, suggesting annual crowds in the range of 100,000.[12] In the twelve months following the dedication of the new corona at the east end of the cathedral in 1219, built to house Becket's severed head, gifts of £702 were deposited, implying approximately 180,000 visitors.[13]

Our present interest, of course, is in those who visited a saint's shrine in hopes of receiving a cure for an illness.[14] The custom of doing so, then as now, reflects two common beliefs: that the special powers ascribed to saints to facilitate miraculous acts of healing were most efficacious at the shrines where their relics lay in repose; and that the saints were especially pleased by acts of adoration that took place at the site of their tombs. To understand the source of these beliefs, we need to examine the ideas people had about how and why they became ill and what they needed to do to become well again.

CULTURAL MEANINGS OF SICKNESS

During the medieval period, illness confronted people with profound religious and moral issues. This is because illness was often not ascribed to germs or organic processes but rather to sin. People fell ill, it was said, because of their sins.

Some examples of medieval reasoning about illness can be found in the writings of the fifth-century saint Gregory of Tours. The medievalist Raymond van Dam cites numerous instances of people coming to Gregory seeking cures (a number of the miracles ascribed to him took place while he was still alive and serving as the bishop of Tours). He mentions the case of a man experiencing paralysis of the hands, which the bishop attributed to his sins. There were couples whose children were born crippled or with epilepsy, or who contracted leprosy. These events, according to Gregory (known for his zeal for keeping the sabbath), were a result of the fact that the parents conceived the children on a Sunday, a saint's day, or another holy day. He mentions a man who yoked his oxen on a holy day and soon thereafter became disabled. In another case a man came to Gregory seeking relief from a throbbing pain in his hand. The bishop ascribed his affliction to his failure to abide by a solemn promise he had made to another man and sworn on a Bible. When a woman complained to him that her hands felt as though they were on fire, he explained that her symptoms had come about because she had tried to hoe her field on the day of a great religious festival. He refers to a man whose hand had become frozen into a fist and explained this malady as a result of milling grain on important festival days. In these and other cases of illness, Gregory's explanation was the same: "Physical afflictions are the direct and inevitable consequence of people's sins."[15]

Ordinary people apparently shared this belief.[16] Others might say of those who became ill that they had insulted a favorite saint, harmed his shrine, or defied the liturgical calendar by working or engaging in other inappropriate activities on a holy day. In one way or another, illness was seen as prima facie evidence of sin.[17]

This view of illness derives from the doctrine of original sin. As a result of humans' fall from grace, Satan gained power over people's bodies as well as their souls. Though certain rituals, such as baptism, could be prophylactic, the only certain way to stay healthy was to attain and remain in a state of grace; the moment a person committed a sin, the devil could enter the body and corrupt it. And because sickness was diagnostic of sin, the way to treat it was to confess transgressions and do penance. Medicines could be effective only if miscreants confessed and asked forgiveness first. The conviction that sin was at the root of all illness helps explain the unconcealed hostility of theologians toward members of the medical profession. For example, the Lateran Council of 1215 discouraged physicians from visiting a patient unless a priest had seen him first. A synod meeting in Paris in 1429 went so far as to forbid physicians from treating patients in a state of mortal sin: absolution was required first.[18] Doctors, it was said, themselves committed a sin by endeavoring to cure bodily symptoms while ignoring the spiritual origins of the patient's complaint.

Because sickness revealed moral failings, those displaying overt signs of illness—especially those with leprosy, skin lesions, paralysis, blindness, deafness, deformity, and mental disorders—became ready targets for stigmatization, ostracism, and marginalization.[19] Illness posed troubling problems not just for the sufferer; it also threatened the community, and not only because of the fear of physical contagion. Aron Gurevich observes: "Medieval man was not an isolated individual facing the world on his own; he was a member of a group in which the moods, sentiments and traditions of his consciousness were rooted."[20] As a result, to quote Jonathan Sumption, "The sins of one were the business of all."[21] Individual and community were one. In consequence, an individual whose sins offended God jeopardized not only his own soul but also the lives of others. God's anger toward the miscreant might lead him to withdraw his protection from the entire community.[22]

Equating sickness and sin also affected the way people regarded miracles. If someone was cured through the intercession of a saint, it was believed that God had forgiven the person her sins.[23] Eamon Duffy explains: "The healing mediated by the saint restored more than health to the sick; it restored them to the community of the living."[24] Not only did a miracle allow the healed individual to return to the community with her reputation restored, but it actually enhanced her social status. As noted previously, accounts of cures taking place at healing shrines, both medieval and contemporary, are littered with references to the new *miraculés* as "sacred protagonists," "religious celebrities," "sacred celebrities," and people granted "ambassadorship to heaven."[25]

Elements of this way of thinking about illness persisted well into the nineteenth and early twentieth centuries at popular shrines. At Lourdes, for example, Ruth Harris reports that "rural pilgrims seemed not to distinguish between *santé* (physical health) and *salut* (spiritual well-being), and in their rites sought to break down the boundaries between the material and the spiritual."[26] Yet the situation of a pilgrim to Lourdes was different from that of a medieval pilgrim. For the *miraculés* of Lourdes, illness carried different connotations.

Suzanne Kaufman aptly describes the early Lourdes pilgrims as "sacred protagonists," people who played the lead role in a grand social drama pitting reinvigorated traditional religious thinking against more recent scientific understandings of illness.[27] Brochures describe the *miraculés* of Lourdes as long-suffering people (mainly women) who, through prayer and bathing in the waters of the grotto, were miraculously cured.[28] But historical research suggests that the real story is more nuanced and interesting. It is true that those who experienced cures were long-suffering in the sense that they had been incapacitated by illness for long periods.[29] But popular propagandistic accounts often fail to mention the ongoing, often intense disputes between these women and their medical care providers—in most cases village physicians. The typical *miraculée* portrayed her physician as indifferent to her suffering. The doctor seems to have encouraged the patient to visit Lourdes simply to get her out of his hair. In some cases the doctor ridiculed the patient's decision as borne of mere superstition. Physicians told the women there was nothing wrong with them, that their illnesses were all in their heads.

Kaufman lists the core elements of the *miraculée's* personal narrative: "A suffering woman of virtue [who] contends with grievous physical misfortune; her hardship . . . compounded by an ineffective, often coldhearted doctor; her cure . . . sudden and instantaneous, defying all natural explanation." *Miraculées* portrayed themselves and were portrayed by others as victims not only of disease but also of incompetent doctors. The medical treatments were depicted as "torture" treatments, regimes to which doctors stubbornly clung until they gave up in the face of overwhelming evidence of failure.[30] Whereas in medieval Europe illness could bring the sufferer into conflict with others in the community, in nineteenth-century Lourdes the conflict was between the sick person and representatives of the new field of science-based medicine.

Joining a pilgrimage to Lourdes led to a dramatic reframing of *miraculés'* personal experience of their illness and how they viewed it. They now saw their long period of suffering as "making sense," holding a cosmic significance. They understood it as part of a divine scheme that would culminate in a miracle cure, part of a spiritual process in which pain was a prelude to salvation. The mythology of Lourdes recast them as figures not to be denigrated and scorned but to be celebrated.[31]

The narratives of the Lourdes *miraculés* fit neatly with a major theme in nineteenth- and twentieth-century Catholic devotional writing. Kaufman quotes the historian Robert Orsi, writing about nineteenth-century Catholicism: "Catholics thrilled to describe the body in pain. . . . There was always an excess in devotional accounts of pain and suffering of a certain kind of sensuous detail, a delicious lingering over and savoring of other people's pain. . . . Devout women, in particular, were reared on popular religious works that dwelled on pain and suffering as the path of spiritual redemption and knowledge of God." Orsi adds: "Indeed, the devout . . . often encouraged the sick to take comfort in the idea that their intense pain and anguish brought them closer to Christ. . . . [T]he more horrendous the physical suffering endured by the women, the more magnificent the cure."[32]

Given this scenario, it should not surprise us that at least some of the conditions for which miracle cures were claimed—at Lourdes, in the modern shrines of Spain and, insofar as one can tell, at the medieval healing shrines we have discussed—have about them a sense of having been stress-induced, perhaps even mixed with elements of hysterical conversion and psychosomatic disorders. Harris describes some of the sufferers as persons "at the margins of disability," people whose conditions are known to have a large psychogenic component. William Christian echoes this view, commenting on the frequency of sudden disabling paralysis, which today is seen as a probable indicator of hysterical conversion.[33]

TAKING TO THE ROAD

The belief that a saint's special powers were most potent at the site of her tomb or reliquary was one motivation for undertaking a pilgrimage, but medieval pilgrims had other reasons, too. For the sick, coping with the problems of stigma and marginality arising from the association between illness and sin could be difficult or even impossible. As Sumption explains: "The world which the medieval pilgrim left behind was a small and exclusive community. The geographic and social facts of life made it oppressive and isolated and, except in the vicinity of major towns and main roads, the chief qualities of human life were its monotonous regularity and the rule of overpowering conventions." This was especially true of religious practices. Each citizen was considered a parishioner of the local church. As such, an individual "'belonged' to it in a very real sense, and lived his whole life in its shadow. There and there alone, he was baptized and married, attended Sunday Mass, paid his tithe and offerings, and there he was buried when he died."[34] The Lateran Council of 1215 attempted to strengthen the parish church's hold on its members by stipulating that all worshippers must receive the sacraments in their local church only, and that every layman should confess his sins at least once a year to his parish priest and to no one else.

Such an environment offered little privacy. The anthropologists Victor and Edith Turner, who have written insightfully on the topic of pilgrimage, term such environments "intimately localized." They state: "For those tied to a given place and a given set of people, small grievances over trivial issues have a way of accumulating over the course of years and morph and harden into major disputes which have a way of fractionalizing the group. Nagging guilts accumulate, only some of which can be relieved through the parish confessional. When such a load can no longer be borne, it is time to take to the road and go on pilgrimage."[35]

In such an environment, redeeming a reputation tainted by illness was challenging. For a solution, one had to travel outside the community, and a pilgrimage to a shrine was the only real option. Pilgrimage in this context served as a highly effective cultural resource. It enabled people to escape for a time from the social world in which they were so firmly embedded and provided them with a mechanism for setting things right.

This way of viewing illness and cure raises an intriguing possibility. If pilgrimage offered a release from the stigma of illness, it could just as easily become an excuse for those wishing to leave for other reasons. In other words, in some cases the desire to escape might have preceded the onset of illness. This idea occurred to me while reading Van Dam's book about Gregory of Tours. He refers to a woman who felt trapped in a dreadful marriage from which she desperately wished to escape. Her eyesight disappeared, and so she went on pilgrimage. There she experienced a miracle cure. On her return, she announced to her husband that the saint to whom she prayed had instructed her to join a nunnery.[36] Similarly, Peter Brown reports that any slave who received a miracle cure was automatically emancipated and became part of the *familia* of saints, to whom he was now exclusively beholden.[37] Thus cultural scenarios associated with illness and miracle cures might have provided an effective exit strategy for those trapped in desperate circumstances.

Joining a pilgrimage thus served a variety of purposes that are neatly summarized in a single phrase by Peter Brown. He speaks about "the therapy of distance," the recognition that what one seeks or wishes for cannot be found or realized in the immediate environment.[38]

Planning the Trip

We tend to associate pilgrimage with springtime, no doubt in part because of the evocative opening passage from Chaucer's *Canterbury Tales:*

> When the sweet showers of April have pierced the dryness of March to its root and soaked every vein in moisture whose quickening force engenders the flower; when Zephyr with his sweet breath has given life to tender shoots in each wood and field; when the young sun has run his half-course in the sign of the Ram; when, nature prompting their instincts, small birds who sleep through the night with one eye open make their music—then people long to go on pilgrimages, and pious wanderers to visit strange lands and far-off shrines in different countries. In England especially they come from every shire's end to Canterbury to seek out the holy blessed martyr St. Thomas à Becket, who helped them when they were sick.[39]

Spring was indeed a popular season for pilgrimages, but it was not the only time. Nilson's data from the cathedral churches at Ely, Hereford, Durham, and Canterbury suggest that the income from these shrines was greatest during the autumn, followed by the spring and early summer, with the least remunerative period being between Christmas and Easter. Finucane concurs, quoting one source to the effect that a popular time for pilgrimage was after the fall harvest.[40]

Whatever the season, a pilgrim did not act on impulse and of a morning, stumble out of bed, decide over breakfast to take to the road, pack a few belongings, and leave. Pilgrimage required substantial forethought and planning. Sumption quotes the advice given by the fifteenth-century

London preacher Richard Alkenton: "He that be a pilgrim oweth first to pay his debts, afterward to set his house in governance, and afterwards to array himself and take leave of his neighbors, and so go forth."[41] Except for journeys of a day or two to a local shrine, permission of various kinds had to be obtained: from the pilgrim's family, from the lord of the manor to which he belonged, and from the village priest. For longer journeys, wills had to be drawn up, signed, and witnessed in case the pilgrim died along the way. Debts had to be settled, provisions made to cover work obligations, and, for the head of a household, decisions taken about how to provide for the family.[42] An itinerary had to be prepared spelling out the route to be followed, the time of year to depart, what form gifts for the saint should take, and the proposed timetable. All of this took time and forethought. To borrow the jargon of modern psychology, it implied a proactive exercise in self-efficacy.

Rigors of the Journey

All but the shortest pilgrimages posed daunting challenges. Going on a pilgrimage could be a complicated and dangerous business, and this fact gave it a distinctly penitential quality.[43] Van Dam describes pilgrimages during the early fifth and sixth centuries to the shrine of Saint Martin of Tours. Travel was mainly on foot and was slow and arduous. Accidents, delays, and bad weather were common, and bandits were a constant danger. A journey of 70 to 120 miles could take weeks, and pilgrimages to the shrine occasionally lasted months.[44] According to Diana Webb, brawls and improprieties were common along the way. Women in particular were vulnerable to attacks both verbal and physical: "Even great pilgrimage churches occasionally had to be re-consecrated because violence, even rape, or bloodshed had occurred within them."[45]

These were conditions commonly associated with relatively modest trips. The difficulties of longer pilgrimages, to locations such as Compostela or Jerusalem, nearly defy comprehension. In his *Pilgrim's Guide to Santiago de Compostela*, William Melczer describes in graphic detail some of the rigors of this particular journey (see map 1). From southwestern France, the distance to Compostela was 1,000 to 1,200 kilometers; from the eastern or northern provinces of France, distances were 1,600 to 2,000 kilometers; and those who began from Germany, the northern countries, or England faced journeys of 3,000 kilometers or more. All the roads leading to Compostela were dangerous and conditions unpredictable. The trails through the mountains of Navarro and Galicia were rocky, often flooded in the spring, and dry and shadeless during the summer and fall. The roads through Castilla were equally hot and parched. "The climatic conditions—heat, cold, storm, rain, snowdrifts, hail—and the natural eco-system that complemented it—flies, insects, and wild boars on the plains; bears and wolves in the mountains—contributed their share to the normal plagues and pains of the route. The four to five hours of marching, the hardly-ever-adequate, let alone satisfying and tasty food, the often pathetic resting and overnight shelter conditions—these alone were sufficient, on a protracted itinerary, to wear out the bravest and the strongest among the pilgrims." He continues: "In the lands and regions to be traversed for weeks and months in a row everything was at every step new, strange, uncommon, outlandish, never before seen, hardly ever heard of, never before practiced: food, drinks, language, landscape, human countenance, custom, behavior."[46]

The pace of the journey depended on the terrain, the weather, and the physical condition of the pilgrims. For the mass of pilgrims who walked their way, twenty to perhaps fifty kilometers was a reasonable average daily march; but there were certainly mountainous stretches through which no more than fifteen kilometers could be traveled in a day. The length and hardships of the journey wore the pilgrims down—especially those who were already ill.[47]

Many pilgrims lived off charity en route.[48] Accommodation at hospitals, hospices, and monasteries was of the humblest nature—often a single sleeping area with one large straw mattress serving as a communal bed, on which ten, fifteen, or even twenty pilgrims accommodated

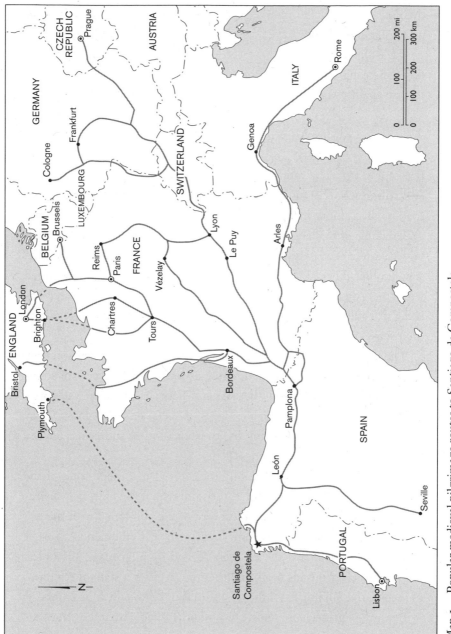

Map 1. Popular medieval pilgrimage routes to Santiago de Compostela.

themselves as best they could, huddled together, warming each other with their shared body heat.[49]

Regardless of the length of the pilgrimage, pilgrims preferred to travel in groups. Marching in company afforded them at least some protection against vagrants, thieves, and other asocial characters.[50]

ON BEING "BETWIXT AND BETWEEN"

If escaping from the intimately localized existence of the typical medieval village was liberating, it could also be disorienting.[51] Taking to the road involved more than simply withdrawing from daily village life and undertaking a challenging journey. People carried with them, albeit unwittingly, a need to experience the same intimacy from which they had sought relief. This need profoundly affected the relationships they forged with others on pilgrimage, as well as with the saints whom they were honoring. It could have profound effects on their state of consciousness and their sense of personal identity as well.

Those who have studied pilgrimage in the modern age, some by participating in such journeys, describe unsettling experiences of ambiguity, of finding themselves "betwixt and between" familiar categories of classification and comfortable places of social embeddedness. They experience an inner void, giving rise to what another author has termed "a yearning for intimate closeness."[52]

This state of yearning is readily transferred to others—one of the principal "others" being, of course, the saint who is the object of veneration. The medieval pilgrims' typical way of life combined with the circumstances of pilgrimage to create an intimacy with the saints.[53] Turner and Turner explain that the escape afforded by pilgrimage allows the pilgrim "to clear out his head, and thereby to enter a state of readiness to receive the full impact of the new [situation] into which he enters."[54]

Because pilgrimage is almost always undertaken with fellow travelers who experience similar needs for intimacy, pilgrims quickly form close bonds. As with any encounter between travelers, the shared experience of being in a strange and challenging environment encouraged medieval pilgrims to develop close interpersonal ties. This experience lent a communal dimension to the veneration of saints. Pilgrims did not approach the saint alone, but rather as members of a spontaneously formed and tight-knit group.[55]

Becoming a pilgrim, then, altered one's state of consciousness. At the same time, the rigors of taking to the road dramatically focused one's attention. The troubles that pilgrims left behind were believed to be largely of their own making, the result of sins committed and unconfessed. The troubles they faced while on the road, though equally daunting, were not the result of their misdeeds but simply part of the journey.[56]

Turner and Turner neatly capture the mindset and identity of the pilgrim: "A pilgrim is one who divests himself of the mundane concomitants of religion—which became entangled with its practice in the local structure—to confront in a special 'far' milieu, the basic elements and structure of his faith in their unshielded, virgin radiance."[57] Pilgrimage induces a liminal state of ambiguity that culminates in a new set of circumstances, new bases of identity and experience based on entirely new circumstances, and being surrounded by others in exactly the same situation.

Confessing

To have any prospect of receiving a miracle, one first had to acknowledge and fully confess one's sins. As Sumption explains, "Without a sincere confession, it was generally agreed that pilgrimage would be worthless." Writing about the modern apparitional shrines of Spain, William Christian explains: "Curing is not a simple matter. At these holy places, health cannot be preserved or achieved mechanically; it must be earned through a state of grace and genuine devotion." And Ruth Harris writes of healing at Lourdes: "Pilgrims felt themselves 'stained' and the journey was to remove the dirty patch on their bodies and souls. . . . Appeasing the saint's animosity or exciting his mercy required giving themselves entirely to the process, best accomplished

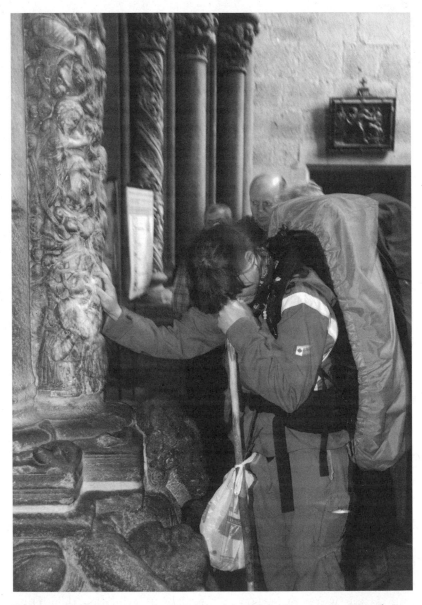

Figure 4.   Pilgrim praying before the statue of Saint James at Santiago de
Compostela. Robert Harding World Imagery/Corbis.

through unquestioning belief, fasting and silence. Once begun, there could be no stopping [or] turning back."[58] Appealing for a cure required pilgrims to fully confess their misdeeds and failings.

It might seem more logical for the pilgrim to have turned to the village priest for confession before departure. However, this course of action carried risks. Despite the supposedly inviolable secrecy of the confessional, local priests often played a key role in spreading gossip and rumors. In addition, as Sumption comments, priests were not universally liked or respected: "A surprisingly large number of pilgrims seem to have left their homes solely in order to deny their parish priest his monopoly over their spiritual welfare."[59]

Pilgrimage, then, entailed elaborate rituals of purification. The pilgrimage way was marked with churches where pilgrims were meant to stop, rest, and confess their sins. By the time he had reached his destination, the typical pilgrim would have confessed repeatedly, performing a final act of confessional cleansing at the site of the shrine itself. Only after doing this could he appeal to the saint in some approximation of a state of grace. At Lourdes today there are fourteen full-time chaplains available to hear confessions, not to mention the priests who accompany pilgrimage groups.[60]

These repeated acknowledgments of one's sins, combined with the harsh conditions of the road, lent a distinct penitential quality to the journey, which in turn affected the relationship between pilgrims and saints.

SHRINES

The changes in mindset that I have described rendered pilgrims more receptive to the experiences that awaited them at the saint's shrine.[61] By the time they arrived at the destination shrine, the freedom, ambiguity, and groundlessness they might have felt on leaving home would have been supplanted by a new frame of mind, organized around religious buildings, images, and rituals.[62]

Local and International Shrines

Pilgrimages varied greatly in length. Those unable to travel at all might walk a labyrinth in or near a local church, such as the one marked on the floor of the nave of Chartres Cathedral. The typical church labyrinth is a complex path inscribed within a circle, traveling from the perimeter to the center and back out again. Lauren Artress, who has written insightfully about the labyrinth, describes it as "a spiritual tool meant to awaken us to the deep rhythm that unites us to ourselves and to the light that calls from within."[63] Her book provides an excellent overview of the labyrinth and its uses throughout history. Though mainly used as a spiritual tool, a labyrinth is occasionally walked by people who are ill and seeking cures.[64]

By contrast, some pilgrimages entailed journeys of considerable distance that would have taken weeks or months and drew pilgrims from far and wide. Among English shrines of the medieval period, Canterbury was the most famous, drawing pilgrims from all parts of England and even from Europe. Ronald Finucane has studied the entries on the 701 pilgrims listed by the monks Benedict and William, who served as registrars for the miracles attributed to Becket. Of those whose origins can be ascertained (fewer than 5 percent of the total), about a third came from outside the British Isles. Of those from Britain, more than half came from villages and towns in southeastern England, near Canterbury; the rest were from more distant locations in Britain, including Scotland and the western counties.[65]

Other shrines drew mostly local visitors. Nine out of ten of those reportedly cured in connection with pilgrimages to Godric's tomb at Finchale, near Durham, came from villages within forty miles of the town. Three-quarters of those who visited Frideswide's shrine and claimed a cure lived within forty miles of her shrine at Oxford, and the great majority of the miracles attributed to visits to Wulfstan's shrine at Worcester Cathedral were experienced by locals.[66] The shrine to Simon de Montfort at Evesham had a more mixed clientele, with roughly equal numbers of pilgrims from the local area and from distant locations.

Finucane has devised a useful metric for determining whether shrines had local, regional, or national renown. He sends a hypothetical pilgrim on his way from a given shrine to his home village and asks at what point half of the villages passed would be home to another pilgrim. For Godric's shrine, the hypothetical pilgrim would have to pass outside a circle with a radius of 15 miles from Finchale before half the villages within the circle contained a miraculously cured resident. For Frideswide's shrine at Oxford, the distance would be 20 miles; for that of Thomas of Cantilupe at Hereford, also 20 miles; and Simon de Montfort's tomb at Evesham, 45 miles. Similarly, most of the recipients of miracles reported in connection with visits to William's tomb at Norwich were locals who lived less than ten miles from the shrine; most of them came from the city of Norwich itself.[67] Though Finucane was unable to compute comparable figures for Canterbury, there is little doubt that it drew pilgrims from a much wider radius than other shrines in England.

Finucane uncovers another important feature of the miracle cures that were attributed to the various shrines he studied (seven in England and two in France). In almost every case, the initial reports of miracles came from pilgrims who lived in the immediate area, but over time, the numbers of local pilgrims diminished, and the numbers from more distant locations increased. William's shrine at Norwich illustrates the pattern. At first, the number of *miraculés* declined sharply beyond a radius of 10 miles from the shrine and dropped to zero at a distance of 50 miles. Over time, however, fewer and fewer locals who visited the shrine claimed to have benefited from it, but the decline of locals was balanced by an increase in pilgrims from more and more distant locations. In 1150–51, for example, the recipients of miracles traveled an average distance of 23 miles; in the period 1151–54, the distance rose to 32 miles; and between 1154 and 1172, it increased to 45 miles, or twice the original average. With each successive translation of his body (his propagandist, Thomas of Monmouth, arranged to have the boy's body exhumed and translated in Norwich several times), the number of cures reported by locals declined. In connection with the initial translation in 1150–51, two-thirds of those claiming miracle cures were citizens of Norwich. By the last translation, the proportion of locals had dropped to less than one-third.[68] This pattern is also reflected in Ben Nilson's analysis of revenues reported by English shrines.[69] In many cases, the number of farther-flung pilgrims gradually declined, too, and eventually the shrine's reputation died out entirely. At Saint Thomas of Cantilupe's shrine at Hereford, 450 miracles were recorded in the shrine's registry. Finucane's study shows that there was an initial burst of reports in 1287, when 160 miracles were reported (mainly by locals), but the number declined to 34 in 1288, 9 in 1300, and only 1 in 1312.[70] After that miracle reports died out entirely.

John Hatcher suggests one of the reasons people might have had for turning to new saints for miracle cures. The notion of sainthood included the idea that God rewarded each saint with a certain number of divine favors. Each time a miracle was granted, therefore, the saint's credit was depleted. As more and more miracles were ascribed to a single saint, people were apt to turn elsewhere for help.[71]

Though the explanations are different, there is a remarkable parallel between the apparent initial efficacy of medieval shrines and a well-established pattern in modern medicine: when new drugs are first introduced, they almost always appear efficacious, but over time their efficacy appears to decline, and newer drugs and treatments come along to take their places (see chapter 7).

As Sumption explains, supporters had to find ways to explain the apparent decline in a saint's powers. In discussing Becket's shrine, one of its registrars, William of Canterbury, reflected that once a saint has performed enough miracles to command veneration, he withdraws gracefully and leaves the task to other, more recently canonized saints.[72] Some of the traditional saints continued to draw crowds on their feast day or in jubilee years; Thomas Becket was among them, but there was no continuous cult as there had been at the peak of his fame in the twelfth century.[73] The loyalty of the masses was spread over an enormous number of minor shrines that commanded attention for a few weeks before relapsing into obscurity and being replaced by others.

Ambience at the Shrine

Detailed descriptions of what actually transpired at medieval healing shrines are difficult to come by. Nilson offers one explanation: "The medieval view seems to have been that everyone knew what happened at a shrine, and therefore it needed no description."[74] The few surviving accounts of medieval healing shrines nevertheless suggest how unusual their environment was.

Every effort was made to evoke the saint's spiritual presence. The architecture of the building and its reliquary or tomb, the iconography, the stained glass, and the use of incense, jewels, and music, were used to create the impression that the saint was present in spirit and therefore available to supplicants. A palpable sense of the saint's latent power was further fostered by housing her relics in a statue resembling her earthly appearance. The aim was to create an atmosphere dense with what Diana Webb has termed "localized holiness," a "hot line" to the divine, or what Turner and Turner describe as a setting "vibrant with supernatural efficacy," a place of contact with other worlds.[75]

Surviving accounts of medieval healing shrines evoke a bewildering mix of calm, serenity, hysteria, and utter chaos. One account describes church of Saint Denis near Paris on the saint's feast day. Its famous twelfth-century leader, Abbot Suger, speaks of crowds so tightly packed that those who managed to enter were soon forced out again. Such crowds could become so unruly that trying to worship the abbey's great relics—a nail from the cross and the crown of thorns—became impossible. Suger notes especially the distress of women "squeezed in by the mass of strong men as in a winepress, (they) exhibited bloodless faces as in imagining death; . . . they cried out horribly as though in labor; . . . several of them, miserably trodden underfoot [but then] lifted by the pious assistance of men above the heads of the crowd, marched forward as though upon a pavement."[76] Events got so out of hand that the monks charged with responsibility for displaying the great relics were forced to flee with them through the church windows.

Sumption provides a composite description of a typical pilgrimage scene based on materials gathered from a number of different medieval shrines. On a saint's feast day, the crowds of the sick, wrapped in blankets or lying on makeshift beds in the basilica, were surrounded by relatives and well-wishers. Because of the crowds, many had to wait for long periods before gaining admission to the church. When relics were not visible for public display, pilgrims instead gathered dust, stones, water, and even scraps of paper that had been in contact with the shrine, then rubbed them on their bodies or ingested them. At the shrine to Gregory of Tours, for example, the sick chewed wax from candles at the site, and some ate the charred wicks. During an epidemic of dysentery in the Loire valley at the end of the sixth century, many of the sick drank water mixed with dust gathered from the tomb of Saint Martin of Tours, and others drank the water that had been used to wash down the sarcophagus in preparation for Easter. Sumption also relates instances in which those who were sick took a splinter from the true cross, mixed it in water, and then drank it. In the eleventh and twelfth centuries, it was common to dip relics in water or wine and give the liquid to pilgrims to drink. At Norwich, pilgrims mixed water with scrapings of cement from William's tomb; and at Reading Abbey, whose most valuable relic was the hand of Saint James, the saint's bones were dipped in water, and the water was either drunk on site or transported in vials to people who were too sick to leave home.[77]

Pilgrims passed entire nights in the nave or next to the shrine in vigils honoring the saint. Those who were sick were carried in on litters, and they were accompanied by helpers and believers who not only assisted them to the altar or reliquary but also supported and encouraged them in making appeals to the saint. Helpers and bystanders were invited to witness and participate in the shrine's pageantry and rituals—a practice that continues at Lourdes—to join in the Magnificat, and to otherwise immerse themselves prayers and devotions.[78] It was during the vigils that miraculous cures sometimes occurred.[79]

Events at contemporary shrines, for which we have eyewitness reports, help us imagine what medieval shrines might have been like. At

Lourdes, for example, processions add grandeur to the pilgrims' visits. The most important of these is the Procession of the Blessed Sacrament. The inaugural procession, held in 1888 under the guidance of Father François Picard, involved an elaborate procession along the newly built esplanade and was led by priests who carried the consecrated host to display to the *malades* and begged God to heal the sick, followed by able-bodied pilgrims.[80] Those who were too ill to walk were transported in wheelchairs or on stretchers to the grotto, where they pleaded to be cured as the sacrament passed before them. In time this procession became the shrine's most important public ritual.

Other practices at Lourdes are still observed to enhance the holiness of the environment. Since its inception, women have always been the main caregivers for pilgrims.[81] Volunteers accompany the sick on the journey by train or coach; others meet them on arrival, tending to their every need in a manner that emphasizes direct physical contact and loving care. Volunteers also help the *malades* prepare for bathing in the sacred waters of the grotto.[82]

Conditions surrounding pilgrimages to Lourdes are, of course, different from those of the medieval period. A transportation system delivers pilgrims to the site, the press is waiting to report any miracles that may occur, and sophisticated commercial enterprises offer various goods and services to pilgrims. Even so, examining how Lourdes became established and what has transpired there since its inception in 1858 gives us some impressions of the spiritual (and commercial) power of these sacred places.

Ruth Harris writes of early practices at Lourdes: "Understanding what took place requires an imaginative sympathy for the psychic and physical world that pilgrimage generated, for the way intense prayer, unabating pain and extreme humility were bolstered by the support of helpers and believers convinced of the ubiquity of miracles at Lourdes."[83] Ruth Cranston writes about "the beauty of the surroundings, the pageantry and ritual of a great church bringing dignitaries and endless caravans of common folk from all over the world. But above

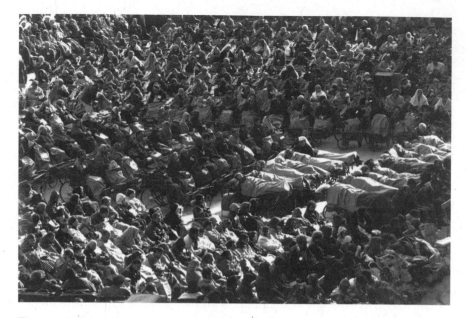

Figure 5.   Open-air mass at Lourdes. Ferdinando Scianna/Magnum Photos.

all, the perpetual prayers, going on day and night, on the part of vast numbers of people—so that the very air is charged and vibrant with it."[84]

William Christian characterizes the shrines he studied in Spain as "energy transformation stations . . . loci for the transformation of human energy for divine purposes" and "major exchange Centers where debts to the divine are paid."[85] Others speak of shrines as "stock exchanges for transactions between the sacred and the secular" and as "dynamic centers at which divine power was concentrated and from which it flowed."[86] And most scholars who write about shrines emphasize another quality they share. Like great cathedrals, they are meant to create the impression of being places where heaven is uniquely present and accessible on earth, an impression that is created not just by their architecture but by other aspects of the environment as well.

People go on pilgrimages for all sorts of reasons, only some of them having to do with illness. But the significance of the miracle cure is

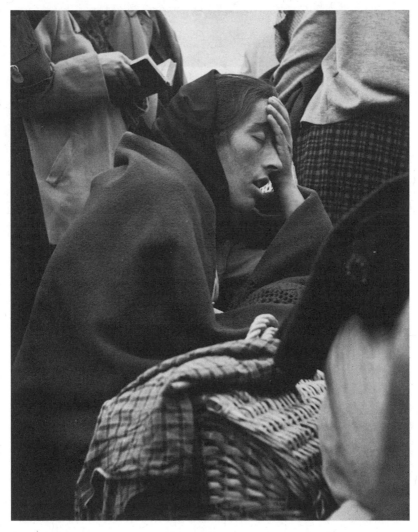

Figure 6.   Pilgrim praying at Fátima, 1951. © Hulton-Deutsch Collection/
Corbis.

its demonstration to the faithful that the divine is indeed present. The occurrence of a miracle cure, or the evidence of such cures—including abandoned crutches, wax models of body parts, and other detritus—enlivens for all visitors the saint's presence in this place, available to them for their own purposes.[87]

Shrines are unique settings of role reversal. Harris explains: "Lourdes, like all healing shines, is a place of special sociological significance for those who are sick and dying. In normal daily life such persons are relegated to the margins of society, ignored, forgotten, often denigrated, invisible. At healing shrines they take center stage. . . . Lourdes made the disgusting elevating and brought the hidden into the open."[88] Conversely, penitents who are sick or in pain often seek to experience suffering, particularly the suffering of Christ. To this end they perform acts of self-torture such as crawling on hands and knees, flagellating themselves and one another, walking barefoot, wearing crowns of thorns, and starving themselves, all in an effort to convey and express their genuine penitence and sense of intimacy with Christ.[89] These acts of role reversal add to the special aura of the shrines—inside-out, upside-down settings that place them apart from the world of the ordinary.

Publicity and Fame

In medieval times, initial word of a miracle cure at a medieval shrine spread by word of mouth. Such events caused tremendous excitement, and as news spread through the town, crowds of locals were drawn to the shrine. The resident clergy would erupt in a Te Deum as observers struggled to see and touch the body of the person who was cured. The situation of the *miraculés* at Lourdes excited similar reactions. Suzanne Kaufman writes: "Pilgrims, on seeing a cure unfold before their eyes, lost all control and converged on the recipient." But visitors to Lourdes stood to gain widespread regional and national fame. The Catholic press of France had a seemingly insatiable appetite for stories of miracles. The coverage invariably included information about who the individual was, details of her condition before bathing in the waters of the grotto, and what happened to her thereafter. The instant local and national celebrity that greeted the new *miraculés* often contrasted sharply with their social standing at home. Those whose names are inscribed in the record books of Lourdes were mostly ordinary, unknown women, usually in their thirties, who came from villages and towns (and, less often, cities) throughout France. Until their cures, their lives had been entirely unexceptional. Most were unmarried and employed in menial, difficult, and debilitating work.[90]

For most, the renown was only temporary, amounting to no more than a headline story in one of the weekly religious newspapers.[91] For others, however, celebrity was more lasting. In connection with major public events such as the shrine's jubilee celebration, marking the twenty-fifth anniversary of its founding in 1872, *miraculés* were invited back to the shrine, where they marched at the head of great public parades wearing special insignia, and their cases were inscribed in the permanent record of cures at the shrine.

As with other shrines, whether medieval or modern, propagandists played a crucial role at Lourdes. In connection with the 1897 jubilee, the *miraculés* selected to participate in the various public events were carefully screened by the Assumptionist Fathers. Through ads in the national Catholic press, the fathers solicited applications from people who claimed to have been cured at Lourdes. These candidates were required to submit certificates from their local doctors attesting to the facts of their illness and recovery, accompanied by testimony from their parish priests. To ensure their participation in the jubilee, the Fathers provided travel grants to *miraculés* of modest means.[92]

The exploitation of these *miraculés* at the jubilee celebration was sometimes shameless. Kaufman describes the behavior of Father Picard, head of the Assumptionist order, who marched with the *miraculés* and exhorted the hundreds of sick pilgrims who were watching: "Behold, your friends, your models. . . . They were once like you, now do as they did. They lay in stretchers, they got up. What is stopping you? . . . Get up!"[93]

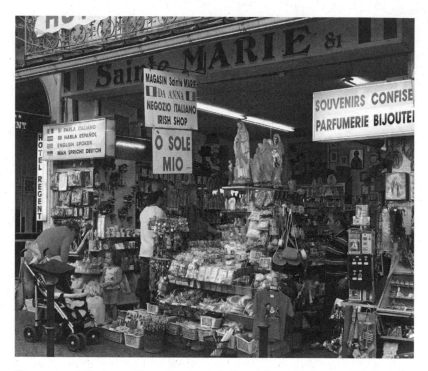

Figure 7.   Gift shop at Lourdes, 2006. © Franz-Peter Tschauner/Corbis.

Commercialism

Healing shrines had the obvious potential to become engines of local economic growth and development. Great pilgrimage sites have always attracted markets. Inns and eateries are required to feed and house pilgrims. Vendors arrive to sell pilgrim badges, packages of dirt and vials of water from springs near the saint's tomb, statues and figurines of the saint, and other souvenirs and religious paraphernalia. Suzanne Kaufman's study of Lourdes, aptly titled *Consuming Visions*, provides a compelling picture of this industry.

At its inception, the potential of Lourdes for generating economic development and profit was scarcely evident. From early on, large crowds were drawn to the site, but these were mainly onlookers curious to witness Bernadette in one of her many raptures. Thus, on March 4, 1858, one month after her first vision, a crowd estimated at seven thousand gathered at the grotto to watch Bernadette as she fell into an ecstasy. By October, national newspapers were providing accounts of her visions, and the local mayor, responding to the appeals of growing numbers of pilgrims, permitted access for informal pilgrimages.[94]

Although the grotto gained increasing attention in the national press, most visitors to the shrine for the first eight years of its existence came from nearby villages and towns and stayed for only a day, or sometimes two. In 1866, however, the local bishop asked a group of monks, the Missionaries of Notre Dame de Garaison, to take over the administration of the shrine. Known more familiarly as the "Grotto Fathers," they were the first to glimpse the shrine's economic potential, and they began to draw up plans to expand the site. They arranged with the regional railway company, the Compagnie des Chemins de Fer du Midi, for a branch line to be built to connect Lourdes with the departmental capital of Tarbes. To promote the idea of a great national pilgrimage, in 1866 they organized a ceremony of inauguration for the yet-to-be-built basilica, which brought nearly fifty thousand pilgrims to the site. Its success prompted them to organize annual pilgrimages thereafter.

In 1869 the shrine gained further national renown when a devout Catholic journalist, Henri Lasserre, published a book titled *Notre-Dame de Lourdes*. His book was inspired by a miracle cure he claimed to have experienced in connection with his visit to Lourdes six years earlier. It told the story of Lourdes by recounting Bernadette's apparitions and the miracle cures people had experienced following immersion in the waters of the grotto. Kaufman characterizes the story as "a tale of rustic peasant spirituality," a theme that resonated with many urban dwellers nostalgic for a peasant culture they perceived as vanishing.[95] The book became a bestseller and, along with the new railroad, helped turn Lourdes into a great national shrine.

The economic potential of Lourdes was further exploited when a Paris-based monastic order, the Augustinian Fathers of the Assumption (the Assumptionists), assumed joint "ownership" of the shrine with the Grotto Fathers. The agenda of the Assumptionists has been described as the re-Christianization of a nation whose main institutions and citizens they saw as alarmingly secular.[96] In Lourdes they perceived a potent weapon in their campaign to restore the power of the Church in France.

The Assumptionists took the practice of annual pilgrimages to an entirely new level. They joined forces with a Catholic women's lay organization—the Association de Notre-Dame de Salut—to raise funds to help underwrite the costs of pilgrimages. They also recruited an order of nursing nuns, the Petits-Soeurs de l'Assumption, to look after the sick pilgrims who came to Lourdes. In 1873 one of their members, Father Vincent de Paul Bailly, began publishing a weekly newsletter for national distribution. Known as *Le Pèlerin* (The Pilgrim), it presented articles about news of recent pilgrimages to Lourdes, including spectacular accounts of recent miracles. It also provided information about train schedules and travel and hotel rates for forthcoming pilgrimages. The head of the Assumptionist order, Father Picard, negotiated with the French railroads for pilgrim discounts on rail fares and also persuaded them to build special train cars with compartments to accommodate travelers on stretchers or in wheelchairs.

Beginning in 1875, the Grotto Fathers and the Assumptionists began working with officials from the village of Lourdes to create an infrastructure capable of handling the growing crowds of pilgrims. Electricity was installed. Old neighborhoods of the village were torn down, wide streets and boulevards were created to accommodate grand processions to the grotto, hotels were opened, a tramway and funicular were built to transport tourists from the hotels to the grotto, a new residence was built for the Grotto Fathers, a shelter was erected to house poor pilgrims, and the basilica whose foundations had been inaugurated in 1866 was now being finished. Kaufman writes that all these changes and more were "intended to transform Lourdes into an attractive and well-functioning sacred city."[97]

Next came myriad commercial and industrial enterprises that supplied goods and services to pilgrims. Boutiques sold votive candles, rosaries, napkin holders, metal cups, and containers of Lourdes water that pilgrims could take home. For those unable to make the pilgrimage to Lourdes, arrangements were made to market containers of Lourdes water in stores throughout France. So ambitious was this program that, according to Kaufman, a government report issued in 1899 estimated that in that year alone, 100,000 bottles of Lourdes water had been sold, generating 60,000 francs for the grotto administration.[98]

A series of guidebooks appeared, aimed at the ever-growing market of Lourdes pilgrims. They presented detailed information about travel, cheap accommodations, and inexpensive places to eat—late nineteenth- and early twentieth-century harbingers of Frommer's *Europe on $5 a Day*. (One source declared that it was possible to make a four-day pilgrimage for less than seventy francs.)[99] The books suggested schedules that would allow pilgrims to make the most of a three- or four-day visit. In advertisements in French Catholic newspapers and magazines, the sponsors emphasized that the town now boasted a number of high-class hotels and grand stores, and that all visitors were welcome to browse the shops and visit the lobbies of the grand hotels.

This advertising campaign points to another goal of the organizers: to appeal to women from the rural villages of France. In the guise of rural piety, it invited women of modest means in rural areas to experience the wonders of modern-day urban and commercial life. Entering the lobbies of luxurious hotels and browsing the aisles of upscale stores acquainted these women with a lifestyle they would otherwise never have known. Those seeking cures for their illnesses, or accompanying others seeking cures, were also offered the chance to enjoy a few days' holiday. Kaufman writes: "This new Catholic pilgrimage provided . . . an alternative mass-cultural experience for Catholics, especially rural women, who now experienced the joys of sightseeing, buying and even people watching in an environment that was sanctioned by religious authority."[100]

Kaufman reports that by the early twentieth century, hundreds of small piety shops lined the two main boulevards leading to the grotto, side by side with large luxury emporiums selling religious articles of every kind. One shop, Maison Puccini, boasted a stock of ten thousand different-sized models of saints. To these offerings were added dioramas, panoramas, and wax museums containing life-sized figures of Bernadette and the Virgin.[101] By the time of another major celebration in 1908, the fiftieth anniversary of Bernadette's vision, Lourdes had become transformed into something like a religious Disney World.

If shrines contain the potential for stimulating commerce, they can also attract the corrupt, the greedy, and the criminal element. This facet of commercialization is illustrated by one famous product offered in shops throughout the town: *pastilles de Lourdes*, lozenges made from sugar and grotto water. The manufacturer proclaimed that even a single drop of grotto water was "powerful enough to cure both suffering body and soul." The Grotto Fathers did nothing to discourage the sale of these confections but did balk at the proposed sale of a liqueur named in honor of the Virgin of Lourdes.[102]

Another instance of fraud at Lourdes involved the sale of grotto water. Francisque Sarcey, an anticlerical journalist, traveled to Lourdes and met with an employee of the shrine, Brother Henri Soubiat, who bottled Lourdes water. The cleric revealed to Sarcey how much money the sanctuary derived from bottling water from the sacred shrine. He also showed Sarcey how Lourdes water could be counterfeited simply by placing lead caps bearing the name of Lourdes on ordinary bottles of tap water. The brother sold them to pilgrims, justifying the practice by explaining that because faith alone healed the sick, it did not matter if the water came from Lourdes or from one's own tap.[103]

Huge crowds of pilgrims also attracted beggars, pickpockets, petty thieves, and unscrupulous merchants touting the magical properties of the goods they were selling. Pilgrims complained of price gouging and harassment, and of feeling unsafe while visiting what had been advertised as a secure and sacred site. More and more, the village of Lourdes took on the character of what Kaufman describes as "a religious fairground or a holiday getaway," warts and all.[104]

CONCLUSION

At the medieval shrine, sickness was equated with sin, and healing with forgiveness; at Lourdes and other contemporary healing shrines, religious interpretations for suffering replaced explanations based on medical science. But visits to shrines during both eras demonstrate a remarkable capacity to inspire hope among the sick and belief in the possibility of a cure. Recent research by biomedical, social, and behavioral scientists into factors associated with illness lends plausibility to the suggestion that these two factors actually helped those who were sick to feel better and in some cases even to recover from their illnesses. Part 2 of this book explains the bases of this claim.

PART TWO

Saints and Healing

CHAPTER FIVE

Disease

Chapter 1 introduces the common forms that illness took during the Middle Ages. In this chapter I examine them in greater detail. I draw on two kinds of sources: studies that describe diseases common in this period, and reports of miracle cures that appear in registers of medieval healing shrines.

No studies of medieval illness employ modern standards of epidemiological research. Instead, we must rely on sources that supply hints and clues, which are often murky.[1] Some of these come from the studies by medical historians cited earlier, and some from medievalists who study the epidemics that periodically swept these societies.[2] Still others come from research that describes patterns of morbidity in contemporary societies whose standards of living, life expectancy, and patterns of economic development approximate those of medieval and preindustrial Europe.[3] By piecing data together from these varied sources, we can develop a rough picture of the patterns of morbidity characteristic of medieval populations.

HISTORICAL STUDIES OF MORBIDITY

Given the short average life span in the Middle Ages, we would not expect to encounter the kinds of diseases characteristic of aging populations today. Heart disease, stroke, many cancers, age-related dementia, osteoporosis, and degenerative diseases of the joints and muscles were comparatively rare. In their place we find a spectrum of disorders characteristic of populations who did back-breaking manual labor, survived on suboptimal diets, lived among vermin, parasites, and animal and human feces, and lacked clean drinking water or adequate protection from the wet and cold.

Such environments are breeding grounds for infectious diseases of all sorts, particularly among people whose immune systems are already compromised by the chronic stresses associated with intimate communal existence, violence, and fear. Upper and lower respiratory-tract illnesses, ear and sinus infections, fevers, dysentery, and other gastrointestinal disorders are rampant. Poor hygiene results in skin diseases of various kinds and contributes to endemic eye infections. Because of poor sanitation, wounds easily become infected and are slow to heal.

The writings of physicians of the medieval period and medical historians are filled with examples of such conditions. Diagnostic manuals make frequent reference to fevers, infections, fatigue, diarrhea, and joint pain. Although the terms used to describe common illnesses are not the ones used in modern medical textbooks, the diseases to which they refer are certainly well-known today. For example, one condition commonly mentioned is the "bloody flux." Its symptoms included watery stools, high fever, cramps, and dehydration: these are diagnostic of dysentery, a condition caused by a variety of infectious organisms found in food and water contaminated by fecal matter. Another condition known by the same name was an infection that caused diarrhea, stomach pains, high fever, severe headache, coughing, and general exhaustion; this would be diagnosed today as typhoid fever. Another common complaint was Saint Anthony's fire, also referred to as "holy fire," "evil fire," "devil's fire," or "saints' fire." This was probably ergotism, caused by ingesting grains infected with the ergot fungus. The terms *lepry* and *lepra* also regularly appear. They refer not only to leprosy but also to other skin disorders, such as itches, rashes, skin lesions, eruptions, flaking, and dryness. Also commonly mentioned is ague, a fever accompanied by shaking chills, high fever, and severe headaches. After a bout of profuse sweating, the headache and fever disappeared. This was most likely malaria, which was chronic in the southern and low-lying areas of Europe and in southern and eastern England. "Tertian fever" and "quatran fever" were also probably types of malaria, with attacks coming in cycles of two to four days. Women might be stricken by "childbed fever," a condition known today as puerperal fever: it is a bacterial infection of the female reproductive organs after childbirth whose symptoms include chills, high fever, stomach pain, and nausea. It can also result in infections elsewhere in the body and can be communicated to the newborn baby. "Red plague," whose symptoms included high fever, chills, blisters, severe headache and backache, and general malaise, is known to us today as the highly contagious viral disease of smallpox. "Winter sickness" was a medieval term for scurvy, a condition caused by vitamin C deficiency.[4] "Dropsy" was what physicians today call edema, a condition in which an abnormally large volume of fluid collects either in the circulatory system or between the cells of body tissue (the so-called interstitial spaces). It has a variety of causes, among them immobility, exposure to extreme heat, excess intake of salt, and kidney malfunction.

DATA FROM MEDIEVAL HEALING SHRINES

The conditions listed above appear with great regularity in the twenty or so registers of miracle cures I have studied from medieval and modern healing shrines. For medieval shrines, my data are restricted mainly to records of healing shrines in England and a few from continental Europe for which English translations from the original Latin texts exist. For later preindustrial and contemporary shrines, my main source of data is the records of Lourdes, supplemented with occasional materials from Chimayo, Fátima, La Salette, Medjugorje, and a few others.[5] The medieval shrines whose registers I have consulted include those of Saint Thomas Becket at Canterbury, Saint Wulfstan and Saint Oswald at Worcester, Edward the Confessor at Westminster Abbey, Saint Cuthbert at Lindisfarne in Northumbria, William of Norwich, Frideswide at Oxford, Saint Osmund at Salisbury, Saint Hugh at Lincoln, Saint Edmund at Pontigny in France, Saint Gregory at Tours, and Saint Hilary at Poitiers. In addition, I refer to research by Ronald Finucane that examines many of the medieval shrines listed above, as well as those honoring Godric of Finchale, Simon de Montfort, Thomas of Cantilupe at Hereford, and, in France, Edmund Rich and Louis of Toulouse. Finally, Ben Nilson's study of cathedral shrines of medieval England discusses the shrines to Saint William at York and Saint Etheldreda at Ely, as well as the shrines at Canterbury, Norwich, Lincoln, Hereford, Durham, Westminster, and Worcester.[6] Although this list is not exhaustive, it seems reasonably representative of shrines for the period.

Unfortunately, the records of these shrines do not provide a detailed inventory of miracles facilitated by medieval saints. In most shrine records, with the possible exception of Thomas Becket's shrine at Canterbury, the actual number of miracles recounted is small and meant to be illustrative rather than exhaustive. Moreover, many reports are maddeningly vague. Their claims for the saint's miracles are nonspecific: "He healed the afflicted"; "he caused the blind to see"; "he made the crippled whole"; "he caused the dead to come back to life." The accounts lack statistics or details that would give us clues to the likely nature of pilgrims' medical conditions. And even when conditions are named, they seldom include descriptions of physical symptoms that would enable us to identify the underlying complaint.

This paucity of detail, of course, limits what can be said about pilgrims' illnesses. It is almost never possible to assert that a pilgrim suffering from a clearly identified medical condition was indeed cured. Moreover, because we know little about the total number of people who actually traveled to various shrines, how many of them were ill, and what conditions they presented to the saint, baseline rates of cure cannot even be estimated, much less calculated with any precision. In evaluating these and other medieval shrines, it is also important to bear in mind

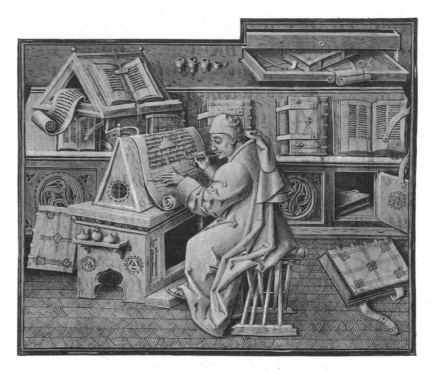

Figure 8. Medieval scribe. From *Miracles de Notre Dame*, 1456. Manuscript Fr. 9198–99. Bibliothèque nationale de France, Département des manuscrits. Courtesy of Art and Architecture Library, Stanford University.

the dubious foundations on which diagnoses of illnesses and evidence of cures were based, and to appreciate that embellishments were added by the registrars in the shrines' books of miracles. This does not mean, however, that we lack any insight at all into the kinds of conditions for which people sought relief through the intercession of the saints.

Records from Thomas Becket's Shrine

The most complete account I have examined of miracles from the medieval period belongs to Thomas Becket's shrine at Canterbury. John of Salisbury (1115 or 1120–80) was a renowned medieval philosopher, historian, and churchman and the author of the famous tome *Policraticus*. He reportedly witnessed Becket's murder in Canterbury Cathedral in December 1170. Later he became treasurer of Exeter Cathedral and then bishop of Chartres. I quote in my prologue his testament to Thomas's miraculous powers to cure. He further proclaims that because of Thomas's privileged place in heaven, "the deformed (are) well-formed; he causes gout and fever to be cured; dropsied and leprous folk he restores; . . . and the mad to return to their senses."[7] How many people were cured of each of these conditions and the details of their sicknesses, John never says. His statements nevertheless suggest an impressive record of healing.

More informative for our purposes are entries made in the two official registers of miracles ascribed to Thomas, recorded by two members of the Benedictine order, Benedict and William, who resided at Canterbury Cathedral during Thomas's lifetime. According to Benedict, most of the early miracles involved people who lived nearby. In one example, Benedict relates how, on the third day following Becket's murder, the news of the archbishop's assassination reached the wife of a knight from nearby Sussex, whom Benedict describes as suffering from "a weakness accompanied with blindness." The woman reportedly cried: "Precious martyr of Christ, I devote myself to thee. If thou wilt restore me the blessing of my lost sight and recall me to health, I will visit thy resting-place to pay vows and offerings." (Benedict does not record how he learned of her condition or obtained the verbatim account of her utterances.) Within half an hour of making her plea, the woman's sight was restored, and within six days she "rose from her bed." Benedict's entry goes on to explain that once cured, the woman reneged on her vow to visit Becket's tomb to give thanks, whereupon her weakness returned. When she renewed her pledge, she again recovered her health and this time promptly went to Canterbury to thank Thomas for her cure.[8]

On the heels of Thomas's martyrdom, Benedict received a flood of reports of miracles, so many that he could no longer keep up with them by himself; hence a colleague, Brother William, was assigned to help him. All of these initial miracles were reported by or on behalf of the persons who experienced them. Only later, as the practice of pilgrimage to Becket's shrine became established as a tradition, did the phenomenon of pilgrimage in search of miracle cures assume its more collective character, as portrayed in Chaucer's prologue to the *Canterbury Tales*.

Both Benedict and William apparently accepted at face value all reports made to them by pilgrims. No serious effort was made to confirm such events. Because of the political context of Becket's assassination, which pitted the crown against the Church, the Benedictine order at Canterbury was anxious to establish the shrine's bona fides as rapidly as possible.[9] For this reason, perhaps, Benedict and William, and the other monks at Canterbury, were willing to believe anyone's word of a miracle cure.

As more reports of miracles poured in, however, the two registrars seem to have become more selective in what they recorded. William, who eventually became the sole recorder of events at the shrine, was able to pick and choose among miracle stories.[10] The tone of the later reports suggests that the shrine was attempting to bolster its claims about Thomas's miraculous powers by showing how exacting their standards were.

DISEASE AND ILLNESS: A KEY DISTINCTION

Most accounts of miracles came from sufferers themselves, a point of some importance for interpreting the accounts that were entered. Modern medicine distinguishes between disease and illness. When medical scientists use the term *disease*, they are referring to what qualified doctors believe is wrong with us; the term *illness* refers to the patient's subjective experience of the disorder. Disease is diagnosed on the basis of signs, that is, measurable changes in bodily functions, such as blood pressure, pulse and respiration rates, temperature, blood chemistry, and the like. Illness is characterized by the symptoms we experience, such as vertigo or headache. Symptoms cannot be observed or measured objectively but only reported and described by the patient.[11]

This distinction between disease and illness is more than merely semantic. A person may be suffering from a disease yet have no experience of feeling ill, and conversely, feel ill while having no disease. A common example is hypertension, a condition that has various causes. Because it can be asymptomatic, people suffering from hypertension, though they may be quite sick and at risk of serious complications, may feel perfectly healthy: they have a disease but no illness. A doctor who diagnoses the condition may place the patient on medications to reduce her blood pressure. A number of these medications have unpleasant side effects, resulting in a situation in which the patient now has no disease but *does* feel ill.

The implications inherent in the distinction between these two terms don't stop here. Studies show that people who are unknowingly hypertensive, when told they suffer from the condition, invoke distinctly different notions about it. Some regard it as an affliction of the heart, others as an affliction of the arteries, and still others as due to emotional upset.[12] These beliefs, in turn, affect the way patients monitor their bodily symptoms. The ones they most notice and report to their doctors are those they consider consistent with the nature and causes of the disease. And, of course, the symptoms they pay the most attention to in effect determine their personal experience of it. In this sense, subjective perceptions shape the answers patients provide when asked how they feel.[13]

The lists of miracles recorded in shrine registers tell us very little about the *signs* of the diseases from which the pilgrims were suffering. What they do tell us about are the *symptoms* they were experiencing. Earlier I made the obvious point that medieval shrines did not have medical authorities on hand to conduct physical examinations or to make competent diagnoses. In most instances, medieval physicians relied on that peculiar mix of the ancient theory of the four humors, ideas and beliefs borrowed from folklore, superstitions, witchcraft, astrology, common cultural understanding, and on-the-job experience.[14]

This is not to say that knowledge-based methods of diagnosis were nonexistent. As Carole Rawcliffe has shown in her recently published work on leprosy in medieval England, physicians knew more about diagnosing this disease than many people today commonly believe. They routinely employed a range of tests, including blood and urine analyses, and had a long checklist of symptoms to help them establish the type of leprosy from which a patient suffered and assess its severity.[15]

Nevertheless, even where medical expertise existed, few could afford the fee for a medical consultation, and those who could were reluctant to subject themselves to the unpleasant, often brutal forms of treatment available. To make sense of their bodily symptoms, most drew on folk wisdom. Thus *illness* determined far more of the experience of being sick than did *disease*. Finucane explains: "In the Middle Ages perception of the illness or healthiness of a given individual was practically a social generalization, whether someone was 'cured' little better than a consensus of opinion."[16] What Benedict and William were recording, then, were symptoms of illnesses, that is, people's subjective experiences of their bodily disorders, tempered by socially constructed ideas about sickness.

Sources of Bias

Because illnesses and their cures were so heavily rooted in cultural understandings, we should not be surprised to discover that people who proclaimed themselves cured employed a somewhat elastic notion of what constituted a miracle. Medieval people thought of miracles as features of everyday life.[17] From this vantage point, it was an easy matter to see evidence of miracles wherever one looked. The result, Finucane explains, is that "the slightest improvement or partial or even temporary recovery was considered a miraculous cure."[18]

Monks who served as shrine registrars also sometimes embellished the accounts of miracles. Although sometimes the monks simply wrote down verbatim what the pilgrims told them, in other cases registrars employed their own terminologies to describe pilgrims' conditions. Those who served as recorders of miracles at shrines had an obvious and deeply vested interest in promoting the efficacy of "their" particular saint in curing illnesses. Such claims, if accepted and widely advertised, could heighten the prestige of the shrine throughout Christendom, bringing monetary benefits.

To demonstrate the local saint's powers and his special privileges in heaven, those who recorded miracles tended to classify reported cases of cure as examples of the same conditions that Christ had miraculously cured during his lifetime. The Bible tells us that Christ healed the leper, restored sight to the blind, and caused the lame to walk, the demented to regain their sanity, and the dead to come back to life. Saints who could perform the same miracles must surely rank among the truly blessed. For this reason, registrars at medieval shrines were inclined to try to make the best fit they could between the medical condition afflicting a pilgrim and one of Christ's miracles. Thus accounts from medieval healing shrines at times display a certain stereotypic quality, in which all types of human ailments are forced into a few standard categories. A minor skin ailment might be classified under lepry, or leprosy. Reports of the cures of the blind comprised not only sightlessness but also eye infections such as conjunctivitis and trachoma, night blindness caused by vitamin A deficiency, and hysterical blindness. Paralysis encompassed not only complete immobility of part of the body but also rheumatic disorders, ordinary joint pain, and even muscle spasms. Cases of revival from the dead might include the recovery of consciousness by those who had fallen into a coma.

Brother Benedict's initial account of cures by Thomas Becket mentions twenty-seven miracles, all listed without explanation or elaboration. There were five cases of blindness being cured; three cures for lameness; two for swelling in the leg or arm; two for a "condition approaching death"; two of fever; one case each of "complaint in head," paralysis, "nocturnal terror," pain in the arm, pain in the jaw, tumor, dumbness, and madness; and five unspecified miracles listed only as "concerning saint's blood."[19]

Brother William's first diary sometimes used different terms to record events, owing in part to occasional acts of literary license and also to the fact that William's record began after Benedict had written his, and therefore presumably does not include all of the miracles that Benedict initially recorded. It too has twenty-seven entries, all but one of which pertain to sicknesses of various kinds; the last refers to a miracle involving the weather. The illnesses include four cases of epilepsy, three of dropsy, three of ulcers, two of festering sores, two of death, and one each of blindness, cough, lameness, intestinal obstruction, "grievous infirmity," "various ailments," "extreme sickness," bleeding to death, disease in the breast, dysentery, piles (hemorrhoids), and swelling of the neck and jaw.[20]

William's entries eventually filled six volumes. Together they identify 426 specific miracles, most of them cures for sickness. For the most part these accounts are no more informative than those in the first volume. Two dozen cases are selected from book 2 to illustrate the point (some may be the same miracles recorded by Brother Benedict and listed above). They include a woman "enormously swollen"; the son of a knight of Pontefract who was "restored to life"; cases of epilepsy, including a nun of Polesworth; a monk cured of "a cough"; an Italian man and his son, a youth from St. Albans, and the wife of the Bishop of Winchester's steward, all cured of "falling sickness"; a lame boy "cured"; a child cured of some unspecified sickness; a priest, one Alan of Lindsay, said to have been cured of "grievous infirmity," who subsequently relapsed but was again restored to health; the cure of a man said to have been bleeding to death; Symon, canon of Beverly, who was restored to life when "all but dead"; Richard, canon of Chichester Cathedral, who was cured of a fistula; Ralph, a clerk, who was cured of a case of "grievous ulcers"; Odo of Aldrington, who was cured of an ulcer on the cheek; William, clerk of Lincoln, who was cured of painful sores in the feet; a nun of Lincoln, cured of a disease of the breast; Ralph de la Saussaie, cured of dysentery; a young man cured of a wound caused by tilting; Adam, a knight near Winchester, cured of a case of piles; Robert of Middleton in Suffolk, and another Robert, a knight of Brompton, both cured of dropsy; Henry of Hythe, a cripple, cured; Reiner of Dodington, restored from seeming death; Cecilia, daughter of Jordan of Norfolk, who was said to have died of cancer and was revived; and Emma of Halberton, whose hand had contracted as a result of working on Whitsun, a holy day, and who was cured after praying to Thomas's relics.[21]

William also recounts an incident demonstrating the power of the placebo effect: a local peasant, who was too ill to make even the short journey from his home to Thomas's shrine in the cathedral, asked a friend to bring him a vial of "Becket water." This was water drawn from a local well, to which was supposedly added a single drop of the martyr's blood, scooped from the floor of the chapel where he was slain. Finding the cathedral closed, and not wishing to disappoint his sick friend, the man drew water from a nearby well and brought it back, telling him that it was authentic. In ignorance, the man drank the water, immediately felt better, and claimed that the saint had cured him.[22]

The lists of miracles from other shrines whose records I have examined read similarly: cures for cripples, lepers, the insane, and the blind; recoveries from fever, tumors, blindness, and paralysis; and returns from the dead.[23] Additional results of my investigation are summarized in the appendix.

DIAGNOSING ILLNESS DESCRIBED AT MEDIEVAL SHRINES

Limited as the information from medieval healing shrines may be, we can still draw inferences about likely diagnoses. A study published in 1986 by the British pediatrician Eleanora C. Gordon attempts to attach diagnostic labels to children's illnesses in the records of several medieval healing shrines. She shows that at least some of the conditions were common, nonfatal diseases of childhood. Her study is based on accounts from the shrines of Thomas Becket at Canterbury, Saint Wulfstan at Worcester Cathedral, Saint Godric at Finchale, William at Norwich, and Frideswide at Oxford.[24]

In all, Gordon identified 216 reports of miracles experienced by children: 125 at Becket's shrine, 27 at Wulfstan's, 25 at Saint Godric's, 22 at William's, and 17 at Saint Frideswide's. She assigns these to five main categories of illness: acute conditions, such as fevers, skin conditions, or eye infections (30 percent); chronic conditions, such as loss of motor functions in the legs, strokes, epilepsy, lameness, eye problems (including blindness, chronic infections, and impaired vision), chronic skin conditions, and bladder stones (29 percent); developmental disabilities, such as inability to speak, walk, see, or hear (20 percent); injuries due to accidents, such as asphyxia due to near-drowning, choking on objects, head injuries, contusions, lacerations, and injuries due to physical assaults (15 percent); conditions attributable to unspecified emotional crises (4 percent); and unspecified gynecological problems in adolescent girls (2 percent).

The illnesses she identified are familiar to modern-day pediatricians and parents of small children. Six children had a sudden illness during which they stopped breathing, became pale and cold, and seemed to have died, which physicians today would label febrile convulsions. This is a condition in which the child experiences a rapid rise in body temperature followed by loss of consciousness and stiffening of various parts of the body, such as the arms and legs. The skin becomes pale, and the limbs begin to jerk. The condition affects one child in twenty, mostly between the ages of one and four.[25]

Eight other cases Gordon examined involved persistent fever and coma. Here Gordon suggests a diagnosis of encephalitis, an acute inflammation of the brain, usually caused by a viral infection. The comatose state into which afflicted children may fall can include loss of pulse, body rigidity, an ashen pallor, and the cessation of breathing— symptoms that could easily have led medieval parents and monks to conclude that the child had died.

Other familiar pediatric conditions include painful swelling of the jaw, the throat, or the neck glands, suggesting tonsillitis, whooping cough, or toothaches; and abdominal pain caused by constipation. She identifies several instances of paralysis as probable cases of childhood stroke. Children experiencing spasms of muscles of the face, neck, trunk, and limbs were probably suffering from Sydenham's chorea, a neurological disorder characterized by rapid, involuntary movements in these muscle groups. It occurs most often in children between the ages of five and fifteen and typically follows acute episodes of rheumatic fever. Other episodes of paralysis and spasms, she believes, were probably cases of childhood polio.

Gordon's study also finds that skin conditions, typically labeled "lepry," were quite common. They included pustules, ulcers, and draining sores—all conditions unsurprising "in an age when good personal hygiene was difficult to achieve."[26] Chronic eye symptoms included swollen lids, together with discharges of blood and pus—symptoms of what we know as chronic conjunctivitis. Ringworm was also common.

Her study suggests that had modern-day knowledge about disease been available during the Middle Ages, many of the illnesses reported by parents to record keepers at medieval shrines would be recognized as self-limiting and the children's recoveries seen as less than miraculous. For example, in the vast majority of cases of febrile convulsions, recovery is spontaneous.[27] Similarly, most children who develop childhood encephalitis also recover spontaneously, typically within about one month.[28] Given the distressing signs of these conditions, however, it is not difficult to understand why medieval parents might have thought their children had died, and why a child's return to consciousness following prayers on her behalf might seem to be the result of a miracle.

Spontaneous recovery from childhood stroke is also common: the patient usually recovers fully over months or years.[29] Sydenham's chorea in most cases resolves within nine months to two years; and even with smallpox, when it is not fatal, the pus-filled blisters simply dry up and eventually disappear within weeks, perhaps leaving permanent scars but no other enduring problems.[30]

NATURALISTIC EXPLANATIONS FOR CURES

Not only children's illnesses but also other symptoms of illness described in the records of healing shrines are familiar to modern-day physicians, and "miraculous" recoveries from them can be attributed to the natural course of the disorder. Some symptoms are known to resolve spontaneously; others ebb and flow over time. Still others are suggestive of conditions that would improve as a result of changes in diet, circumstance, and hygiene associated with taking to the road. In every case, even though the improvements in a pilgrim's health had nothing to do with divine intervention, the saints got the credit.

Self-Limiting Conditions

No one has made a study of adult disorders comparable to Gordon's study of pediatric illnesses and cures.[31] But if we look at the conditions described in the shrine registers, many are recognizable as self-limiting. Examples include infectious disorders, particularly those of the eyes, skin, and sinuses, and superficial injuries; respiratory illnesses such as colds and the flu; headache; and intestinal disorders of various kinds. In such instances it is understandable why some people concluded that the saint had cured them. As they began to recover after leaving home on pilgrimage, they erroneously ascribed the improvement to the saint, not realizing that the conditions from which they were suffering would eventually have cleared up of their own accord in any case.

Precise estimates of the proportion of all illnesses that are likely to be self-limiting are elusive. One website, Patient UK, lists some 332 common conditions that physicians today regard as self-limiting. The term might well apply to a large proportion of the conditions pilgrims presented at healing shrines. Both Finucane and Sumption take the view that the majority of "miraculously cured" illnesses were self-limiting.[32] I am less certain about this, but given what is known about the kinds of illnesses that were endemic in medieval populations, I agree that the proportion of such disorders would have been high.

Chronic Conditions

Another category of common ailment is chronic disorders whose symptoms come and go. Arthritic and other forms of joint pain are examples.[33] Most arthritis sufferers experience alternating periods of great discomfort and mild or no discomfort at all. This pattern can easily cause the sufferer to commit the same attribution error that arises in cases of self-limiting illness: post hoc, ergo propter hoc (after the fact, and therefore because of the fact). People suffering from chronic illnesses are likely to become most motivated to do something about their pain when they feel least well, and are likely to attribute any reduction in pain to the treatments they have received, rather than to the natural ebb and flow of the condition.[34] When the "treatment" involved joining a pilgrimage to a healing shrine, sufferers may have concluded that they felt better because of their pilgrimage and not because the condition had lapsed into a dormant phase or healed of its own accord.

Changes in Circumstances of Living

Some conditions could have been cured by the changes of environment and diet associated with taking to the road. Malnutrition is a principal cause of diminished immunity, with a corresponding susceptibility to infections, and would have been more prevalent in winter, when diets were limited in both calories and micronutrients.[35] Pilgrimage often occurred in late spring. In most years, springtime brought fresh supplies of leafy green vegetables rich in vitamin A and fruits and vegetables laden with vitamin C, both of which would have helped to alleviate edema, night blindness, dry eyes, scurvy, skin lesions, muscle pain, and muscle spasms.

In addition to the more healthful springtime diet, the travel associated with pilgrimage probably had its own health benefits. Fresh air,

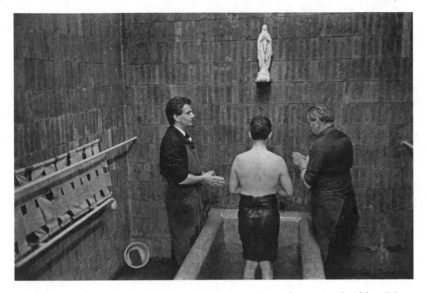

Figure 9.   Pilgrim being immersed in waters at Lourdes, 1987. © Abbas/Magnum Photos.

direct sunlight, and clean drinking water all would have helped alleviate the symptoms of a range of illnesses. The practice of bathing in waters drawn from wells and springs at or near the shrines may also have conferred health benefits, as may have rubbing the skin with mud using dirt from near the saint's tomb.[36] Water from nearby springs would have helped to irrigate wounds and infections, and mud that contains high concentrations of retinoids (a class of compounds chemically related to vitamin A) heals a variety of dermatological conditions, including skin lesions and even some forms of skin cancer.[37]

Other conditions probably healed simply as a result of leaving the environment that was causing them to fester. For example, living in enclosed, unventilated, unheated quarters shared with farm animals probably aggravated eye infections, skin conditions, and respiratory infections. Freed of these unsanitary conditions, and fortified by an improved diet, the body would have become better able to fight off disease. Moreover, research shows that overcrowding can not only spread contagious diseases but also cause elevated blood pressure and various other kinds of stress reactions.[38] These and other negative effects are substantially attenuated when subjects move to less crowded environments, especially if they feel that they have some control over noxious stimuli. Leaving the enclosed nature of daily life in a medieval village to join in pilgrimage might well have had both physically and psychologically therapeutic effects.

CONCLUSION

Simply leaving home and taking to the road generally brought improvements in diet, changes in daily routines, improved conditions of hygiene, and exposure to fresh air and sunshine. Any of these changes could plausibly explain why people might have gained relief from at least some of the conditions from which they were suffering. These changes in circumstances, and the fact that many conditions were self-limiting, provide important clues for understanding why people came to place so much confidence in the healing powers of the pilgrimage.

But this is not the full story. Some accounts of cures are not readily explained by environmental factors. I believe it is possible to construct a more robust narrative about the experience of illness in the medieval and the early modern periods, one that supports the widely held belief that appealing to saints could result in genuine relief of symptoms of bodily illness.

The narrative that follows is organized around three themes: the features of daily life that contributed to illness, and how relief from them could facilitate recovery (chapter 6); why belief in the healing power of saints and the practices in which people engaged to access this power helped to ease their suffering, and in some instances may have actually cured them (chapter 7); and how cultural and religious beliefs structured the ways people experienced their illnesses and led them to engage in actions that might have benefited their health (chapter 8).

CHAPTER SIX

The Role of Stress in Illness

I have described how stress-filled, fearful, and despairing life could be during the preindustrial era, especially for those who became ill and were shunned and isolated. Recent studies of health and illness suggest that social and emotional difficulties are among the root causes of many illnesses, and aggravating factors in others. This chapter examines four social factors directly related to the onset, course, and outcome of illnesses in contemporary populations. Research demonstrates that two of them—stress and emotions—are directly related to the onset of illness, and two others—shame and social isolation—can exacerbate existing illnesses. Because we lack clinical data for the medieval period, we cannot say, of course, that these factors were singly or collectively responsible for anyone's illness. But what we know about the circumstances of daily living and the role that social, situational, and psychological factors play in illness suggests that they contributed significantly to high rates of morbidity.

PSYCHOLOGICAL CAUSES OF ILLNESS
Stress

A mountain of research studies have confirmed the role of stress in the onset of various medical conditions, including those that afflicted people

of the medieval and early modern periods: infectious disorders, tuberculosis, influenza, upper respiratory-tract illnesses, herpes, rheumatoid
arthritis, joint inflammation, psoriasis, and bronchial asthma.[1] Studies
identify stress as a major risk factor for the onset of psychiatric disorders,
including the expression of psychosomatic illnesses: these can include
burnout, anorexia nervosa, depression, bipolar disorder, chronic fatigue
syndrome, asthma, neurodermatitis, and post-traumatic stress disorders.[2] Stress is also a major risk factor for cardiovascular disease, heart
attack, and stroke, and can aggravate and accelerate the onset of cancer,
systemic lupus, multiple sclerosis, ulcerative colitis, and Crohn's disease.[3]

The exact role of stress in illness is only now beginning to be understood. One widely accepted hypothesis posits that stress increases
the body's allostatic load.[4] Allostasis refers to our body's tendency to
increase or decrease the rate of certain vital functions to achieve a new
steady state in response to external challenges. The allostatic systems in
the body—principally the cardiovascular, endocrine, and immune systems—act to protect us from attack by external agents, but their protection is short-lived. In the long run, physiological responses to stress
result in bodily wear and tear that causes ongoing damage and promotes
disease. Thus persistent stresses can lead to the development of an illness, hasten its onset, and worsen its effects.

Stress can impair the efficiency of the body's immune system, a
complicated set of bodily structures and processes whose function is to
identify and destroy foreign agents such as viruses and malignant cells,
and to facilitate the repair of damaged tissues. Anything that diminishes
the immune system's functioning renders the body more susceptible to
invasive agents. We now understand that many of the illnesses suffered
by medieval and early modern people, especially infectious disorders
and parasitic infestations, occurred because their immune systems were
weakened or compromised.[5] Stress-related suppression of the immune
system has been found to increase susceptibility to the common cold
and the severity of cold symptoms in adults and children alike. Upper
respiratory-tract infections are commonly preceded by one or two weeks

of high levels of perceived stress or an unusual frequency of minor life difficulties. The persistent stresses associated with everyday life during the Middle Ages may have rendered populations vulnerable to infections and other illnesses. It seems equally plausible to suggest that once an individual was removed from exposure to these sources of stress, the toll on the immune system would lessen, and her ability to ward off disease would improve.

Emotions

Studies of the role of emotions in causing illness offer additional insights into the experiences of people of the preindustrial world. The link between negative emotions and poor health is a powerful one. Studies find that people who tend to inhibit the expression of emotions have generally poorer health than those with less repressive, inhibited styles of coping. Strong relationships have been found between anger and hostility and the incidence of coronary heart disease, cancer, and arthritis. Equally powerful relationships have been found between extreme sadness, such as that of bereavement, and illness, including heart disease and cancer. Persistent states of high anxiety and fear are also associated with high levels of asthma, ulcers, and headache.[6] And there is now compelling evidence linking pessimism and hopelessness to ill-health and a positive outlook to good health.[7] Optimistic people generally live longer and enjoy better health than those who are pessimistic, and optimists are less susceptible to viral infections such as the common cold. The relationship of emotions to the onset of illnesses is surprisingly strong. In the case of coronary heart disease, for example, the effects of anger and hostility are at least as significant as those attributed to cigarette smoking, high blood pressure, and high serum cholesterol.[8]

Emotional states may affect health in the same ways as stress does. Negative feelings result in physiological changes that adversely affect the immune system as well as our nervous, cardiovascular, respiratory, endocrine, and muscular systems. Individuals who are hostile and prone to anger show larger stress-related increases in blood pressure, heart rate, and production of stress-related hormones than those who are not. In addition, dysphoric mood states such as acute hopelessness and unhappiness can suppress immune functions.[9] Other studies have shown that expressing negative feelings that have previously been suppressed can directly improve immune-system functioning. Psychotherapeutic interventions that effectively treat dysphoric mood have the same effect. Furthermore, the return of depression after successful treatment is often accompanied by the recurrence of illness.[10]

This research suggests that prolonged feelings of fear, anxiety, anger, and hopelessness can cause, worsen, and prolong illnesses, especially those in which the immune system is implicated. Conversely, the arousal of optimism and hope can boost immune-system functions and improve physical health. Going on a pilgrimage offered sick people the prospect of relief from their suffering, providing a powerful antidote to persistent hopelessness and despair. These positive emotions would have strengthened their immune systems, thereby helping their bodies to fight disease.

SOCIAL FACTORS IN ILLNESS
Shame

Because sickness was equated with sin, sick people were often targets of public shaming. Recent research by Sally Dickerson, Tara Gruenewald, Margaret Kemeny, and others has identified a number of pronounced physiological effects associated with intense feelings of shame (and other negative emotions), including stimulation of proinflammatory cytokine activity and increased secretion of cortisol into the bloodstream. In the short term, these physiological responses are adaptive; however, as with persistent stress, repeated or prolonged experiences of shame place individuals at risk for illness and can worsen existing conditions. Chronic or persistent activation of the proinflammatory cytokine network has been shown to suppress the immune system, impeding the body's ability to fight cardiovascular disease, HIV infection, and rheumatoid arthritis. In principle, the same mechanisms may be implicated in any illness involving suppression of the immune system.[11]

This research on shame points to an intriguing conclusion: the practice of going on pilgrimage, with its promise of a miracle cure, could act as a potent antidote, neutralizing the insidious physiological effects of prolonged feelings of shame. If a person began to feel better and interpreted this recovery as a sign that his sins were forgiven, the added burden of shame would be lifted, and the immunosuppressive reactions in the body would decrease. For this reason, participation in pilgrimage might well lead to an improvement in an individual's health and sense of well-being.

Social Support

Shame and ostracism lead to social isolation, which can have profound adverse health effects. Research documents the importance of social-support networks in determining when people become ill; how sick they become; and whether, when, and how they recover. The term *social support* refers to the emotional, material, and social resources provided to individuals by family, friends, and neighbors.[12] Loneliness, weak social support, conflict-ridden personal relationships, and the loss of loved ones can contribute to illness, including specific disorders such as infectious diseases and cardiovascular diseases.[13] Once again, the vector linking social isolation to illness appears to be the immune system. For example, Cohen and his colleagues have shown that rates of infections and illness are more than four times greater among those with limited social networks than among people who enjoy strong social networks. One study on mortality due to coronary heart disease estimates the effects of a lack of social support to be comparable in magnitude to the effects of smoking.[14]

Social-support networks affect not only the onset and course of illnesses but also the outcome. Women with high levels of social support experience fewer complications during pregnancy and have higher rates of successful births. The reasons for this relationship are a topic of continuing investigation. Social support is also associated with lower rates of disability and depression in people with diabetes, and higher rates of compliance in patients on renal dialysis. Among people with cardiovascular disease, mortality rates were lower among those who had at least one close confidante. A study of elderly patients found that patients with poor social support were more likely to die in hospital within six months of a heart attack, even after controlling for the severity of the cardiac event and other risk factors.[15] Other studies demonstrate that social support enhances recovery from medical procedures. For example, a 1995 study of 40,820 patients admitted to a university hospital in Ohio found that unmarried surgical patients tended to stay longer in the hospital than married patients and had a higher risk of dying in the hospital.[16]

Based on these research findings, it seems plausible to hypothesize that the absence of social support exacerbated illnesses among people in medieval and early modern communities. This factor too is related to the equation of sickness with sin and the resulting stigmatization and marginalization of the sick. Such beliefs would have deprived an ailing person of networks of support just when they were most needed. Going on pilgrimage would have reversed this process by placing previously marginalized people in the company of other pilgrims, a society of equals on a common quest for a miracle.

If social isolation has a deleterious effect on emotional well-being and physical health, so too, ironically, does too much closeness. I have explained that the average household consisted of a married couple and their three children living in a one- or two-room hovel. Research shows that living under crowded conditions like these heightens irritability and hostility, provokes aggression, and increases conflict among family members. Such emotions have pronounced physiological effects, such as elevating blood pressure and certain hormone levels, which, if prolonged, are damaging to health.[17]

CONCLUSION

The lines of research I have identified support the conclusion that the stressful conditions of existence for most people during the medieval and early modern eras, the emotional turmoil these conditions caused, and the social isolation resulting from stigmatization of the sick together could have created the health equivalent of the perfect storm, hastening the onset of illness and increasing its severity because of the adverse effects on the immune system. Venerating saints through the institution of pilgrimage offered an escape from the circumstances that created these emotions, alleviated despair, and gave rise to hope. These positive feelings are central to the topic to which I now turn, the role of belief in healing.

CHAPTER SEVEN

Belief, Hope, and Healing

In matters of health, nothing is more fundamental to the practice of appealing to saints than hope and belief: the hope that cures for illness are possible and the abiding conviction that saints can facilitate them. Indeed, in the absence of belief—in God, in the possibility of miracles, in the existence of saints, in their special influence with God, and in their presence on earth—turning to a saint for help in curing an illness makes no sense at all. Among the faithful, it is belief that kindles the hope that they may become well.

Belief also figures prominently in the practice of modern medicine, powerfully influencing how people respond to treatment. Various terms are used to refer to the role of belief in healing today. The most familiar ones are *placebo* and the *placebo effect;* others include *expectancy effects,* the *meaning response,* the *belief effect, nonspecific therapeutic effects,* and the *mind-body connection.*[1] All these terms refer to an impressive and continuously expanding body of research showing that people's beliefs about how they will be affected by treatments can influence how they respond physiologically to them. Even a treatment that is inert or sham, if it is represented by the practitioner as effective, may produce improvements in the patient's condition. These effects, of course, do not apply equally to all illnesses and forms of treatment, and often the placebo effect does not lead to permanent cures. But crucially, belief, as a type of placebo, can temporarily alleviate the pain and suffering that accompany virtually all illnesses.

The placebo research of greatest interest for our purposes is the study of relief from pain—the so-called "placebo analgesia" effect—but there is also evidence of placebo effects for inflammatory reactions associated with pain, skin conditions, injuries, stomach ulcers, depression, anxiety disorders, and even spasms associated with Parkinson's disease.[2] Most studies detect no independently measurable effect of placebos on actual signs of illness, but there is compelling evidence that patients' beliefs about the sham treatments significantly influence how they feel. Placebos may not help people get well, but they can certainly help them feel better.

The beliefs associated with medieval and early modern healing shrines and those associated with recent clinical studies of placebo effects are, of course, radically different. But they do share one feature: the belief that the proposed intervention holds the promise of relief. This similarity led me to wonder what light, if any, modern-day research on the placebo effect might shed on the events that took place at healing shrines.

MODERN PLACEBO STUDIES

One authority defines the term *placebo* this way: "A pharmacologically [or physiologically] inactive substance that can have a therapeutic effect if administered to a patient who believes that he or she is receiving an effective treatment."[3] The aim of placebo research is to discover whether belief alone can have either subjectively perceivable or objectively measurable physiological effects, to learn whether these effects determine how people respond to treatment, and, if they do, to try to understand how beliefs affect the body in ways that promote healing or result in the relief of symptoms.

A swirl of controversy surrounds research on the placebo effect. There are those who conclude that people's beliefs about the likely effects of their treatments powerfully affect how they will respond. Others are skeptical, countering that studies attempting to document the placebo effect are flawed, or that results can be explained more straightforwardly by recourse to well-established principles of natural medicine.

Regardless of this difference of opinion, placebo studies report some astonishing results. For example, studies published in respected, refereed scientific journals report that people who unknowingly receive sham surgical procedures for treatment of knee pain do about as well as those who receive actual procedures; that people given placebos for food allergies are able to tolerate the foods to which they are allergic; that dermatologists are able to eliminate warts simply by painting them with a brightly colored dye and assuring patients that the warts will disappear; that inert substances given to patients for pain relief appear to ease discomfort; that people with stomach ulcers who are given placebos respond just as well as those who receive actual medications; and that people suffering from angina, when treated with sham surgery in which incisions are made but nothing else is done, do about as well as those on whom standard surgical procedures are performed. To deepen the mystery, these and similar effects occur not only when the patient given the placebo believes it to be a real treatment, but also when health-care providers themselves are misled into believing that the inert or sham medications and treatments they administer are real, independent of what the patients may know or believe.[4]

Here I describe two studies that illustrate these findings, chosen from a long list of similar studies. The first measures patients' responses to sham treatments; the second studies the effects of health-care providers' beliefs on the patients to whom sham treatments are given.

Effects of Beliefs Held by Patients

In 1996, the psychologists Guy Montgomery and Irving Kirsch studied people's responses to pain. The subjects (a group of volunteer college students) were told that the researchers were testing a new anesthetic called trivaricane, which had been shown in preliminary studies to show promise for controlling pain. The substance they were given was entirely inert—nothing more than a concoction of iodine, oil of thyme, and water, mixed together to make it look and smell like a "real" medicine. It was displayed to subjects in standard medicine bottles, conspicuously labeled "Trivaricane," with the added phrase "Approved for research purposes only." The experimenter who administered the drug wore a white lab coat and rubber gloves, which subjects were told were necessary to prevent exposing the experimenter to the drug. The experimenter applied the drug to one of the participant's index fingers, allowed a few moments to pass to "give the drug time to work," and then applied a pain stimulus to the index fingers on both hands. The subjects were then asked to rate the pain's intensity and unpleasantness on each finger. They reported that the intensity of pain and the degree of unpleasantness they experienced were significantly lower on the index finger that had been treated with the substance, indicating that the mere belief that the medication had analgesic properties was enough to make it effective.[5]

Beliefs Held by Care Providers

Another study, from 1985, showed that beliefs held by care providers appeared to induce placebo-like responses in those they treat, independent of the beliefs their patients may have held about the treatment they were given. In this experiment, the British researcher R. H. Gracely and his colleagues enrolled sixty people in a study of pain.[6] All of them were having wisdom teeth extracted, and they were told that to control pain they would be given one of four treatments: a placebo, an injection of naloxone (a drug known to counteract the effects of opioids), an injection of fentanyl (a commonly used opioid analgesic), or no treatment at all. Those receiving the placebo were told that the injections they received might reduce the pain or have no effect on it. Patients given naloxone were told they might experience an increase in pain or no difference at all, and those who were given injections of fentanyl were told they might expect to experience a reduction in pain or no difference at all. These conditions were created to test the effects of different expectations on patients' responses. However, Gracely and his colleagues were more interested in studying not what the patients believed, but what the clinicians administering the drugs believed. In the first phase of the study, the dentists and nurses who administered the medications—but not the patients—were told that fentanyl (i.e., the known analgesic) was unavailable. Thus, the clinicians believed that none of the patients could be given fentanyl, even though the patients had been led to believe that use of the drug would be part of the experiment. In phase 2, which began a week later, clinicians were told that fentanyl was once again available, so that some patients to whom injections were being given would now be receiving the true painkiller. The study analyzed the responses to pain of the patients who had actually received a placebo in both phases. The researchers found that pain levels following injections of a placebo in phase 2 of the study (when clinicians believed some patients were receiving a painkiller) were significantly lower than reported levels of pain in phase 1. Because the two placebo groups differed only in the clinicians' knowledge of the range of possible treatments, the results can only be explained in terms of the knowledge held by the dentists and nurses administering the injections, not what the patients thought they had been given.

Other Placebo Studies

Other studies testing different aspects of the placebo effect have yielded equally striking results. R. Barker Bausell offers a succinct summary: "There is at least some evidence (1) that administering a placebo more frequently will produce better outcomes than administering the same placebo less frequently, (2) that some pill colors induce greater placebo effects than others, (3) that placebos in capsule form are more effective than those constituted as pills, (4) that bigger placebo pills are more effective than smaller ones, and (5) that injected placebos produce stronger effects than orally ingested placebos."[7] Daniel Moerman writes: "Large pills work better than middle-sized pills. Blue pills make better sleeping pills than pills of other colors. Four inert pills work better than two. Pills work fine, but shots work better. Surgery works better yet. . . . The form of medical treatment, not just its content, can have a dramatic effect on human well-being."[8]

We might suspect that people who are the most prone to engage in wild imagining or to be influenced by others will respond most dramatically to placebos. Surprisingly, studies designed to test this hypothesis show that the psychological characteristics of recipients do not seem to affect responses to placebo treatment.[9]

One finding of placebo research is in a sense obvious: for sham treatments to work, people must be aware that something has been given to them. The same is not true for active pharmacological agents. A comatose patient who receives medications for, say, anemia will respond to the drugs despite having no conscious awareness of receiving them. A meta-analysis by Andrew Vickers of thirty-three studies of the use of acupuncture supports the claim that patients must be aware of undergoing a treatment if they are to perceive an effect.[10] In four of these studies, the treatment was administered to the patients after they had been anaesthetized.[11] In these cases the acupuncture was only equal to, or less effective than, no treatment. In twenty-seven of the remaining studies, in which patients were awake and alert when the acupuncture was performed, the treatment produced results that were significantly better than no treatment. This suggests that for a placebo treatment to produce results, you have to know that you had it.[12]

Many other placebo studies reinforce the point that our beliefs about the treatments we receive affect how we respond to them.[13]

Criticisms

The conclusions of placebo studies are striking and may explain why some people who appeal to saints experience improvements in health, perceived or real. The studies support the hypothesis that belief in the healing powers of saints is an expression of the placebo effect.

However, placebo research is not without its critics, some of whom identify a problem with the way many placebo studies are designed. One that critics point to as flawed is a study of sham surgery. In 2002, the orthopedic surgeon Bruce Moseley and some of his colleagues set out to investigate the effectiveness of knee surgery by comparing long-term outcomes among people who had received actual surgical operations on their knees with those among patients who had had sham surgery.[14] The study reports that people who were led to believe that they had undergone arthroscopic surgery but actually had not (following anesthesia, surgeons simply made small incisions and immediately sutured them up) were found six months later to be doing as well and experiencing as much relief from joint pain as those who had the received the surgery.

This study resembles many other placebo studies in the sense that it compares outcomes between two randomly assigned groups of subjects—those who receive treatments considered to be appropriate and effective for the condition in question and those who are led to believe they are receiving the same drug or procedure but in fact do not. The degree of the placebo effect is then inferred by comparing outcomes for the two groups.

Critics point out that this type of study fails to take into account the self-limiting nature of many illnesses.[15] (It has been said that if you treat most illnesses they will go away in about a week's time, but if you let them alone they will probably disappear in about seven days!) If we are to accurately gauge whether the placebo effect is genuine, a third group must be added to the study: subjects with the same condition who receive no treatment at all. Without considering the experiences of a no-treatment control group, critics argue, researchers have no way of knowing whether the ostensible placebo effect is due to anything other than spontaneous remission or the natural course of the condition. Among the patients in the Moseley study, some people with arthritic knee conditions that went untreated might, over a six-month period, have recovered naturally. To determine the true extent of the placebo effect, we would need to compare the rate of spontaneous improvement shown by those receiving no treatment with the reported improvement among the placebo group. And, critics argue, when we do this, some (but not all) of the evidence for the existence of the placebo effect for certain kinds of conditions becomes suspect.[16]

This criticism first came to light in a paper published in 2001 in the *New England Journal of Medicine* by two Scandinavian scientists, Asbjørn Hróbjartsson and Peter Gøtzsche. They performed a meta-analysis of 130 placebo studies that included both a placebo group and a no-treatment group. Of these, 114 provided data permitting proper comparisons between the placebo and the no-treatment group. They pooled the results of these 114 studies and concluded that, except for studies where results showed relief of pain, there was scant evidence that placebos had any powerful clinical effects (or even subjectively perceived effects) compared with no treatment at all. In certain cases, when we take into account the natural course of an illness among people who have received no treatment of any kind, the placebo effect evaporates.[17]

Placebo and Analgesia

Hróbjartsson and Gøtzsche's study brought a degree of much-needed rigor to placebo studies and interjected an important note of caution into discourse about it. But it does not negate the findings of *all* the studies I have reviewed. Most important for our purposes, the qualification does not apply to studies of placebo analgesia. Properly controlled studies of patients' responses to inert pain medications yield evidence of a significant placebo effect. The studies that Hróbjartsson and Gøtzsche analyzed show, for example, that headaches, postoperative pain, and sore knees can all be relieved by what amount to different versions of sugar pills. Whatever else we might conclude about placebo effects, it does appear that belief alone can be highly effective in the treatment and relief of pain.

Findings regarding analgesia are, of course, directly relevant to understanding the experience of those who pray to saints for miracle cures. Most human diseases cause pain and discomfort. These studies may help us identify a mechanism for the healing effects experienced by people who go on pilgrimage to seek relief from pain.

Studies of placebo analgesia that have included no-treatment groups in their design show that both the experimental group and the placebo group do significantly better than the no-treatment group, indicating that the effect is real.[18] In addition to Gracely's study demonstrating the effects of clinician's beliefs on analgesia, another study offering evidence of dental placebo analgesia was conducted by two researchers (one aptly named "Hashish") on patients who were ostensibly being treated with ultrasound to reduce postoperative pain following tooth extractions.[19] Unbeknownst to either the dentist or the patient, in half of the cases the machine was deactivated (which was possible because ultrasound treatment is invisible and inaudible). Patients were told that the ultrasound equipment would be used to massage their jaws to reduce pain; following treatment, the patients were asked to indicate their level of pain on a scale ranging from "no pain" and to "unbearable pain." The researchers compared the treated groups (i.e., both those who received actual treatment and the placebo group) to a control group of patients who received no treatment at all. The treated groups reported experiencing a significant reduction in pain regardless of whether the machine had been switched on. Those receiving sham massages of the jaw with the machine turned off showed the same level of pain reduction as those who received the proper treatment. Additionally, evidence from this study shows that the effects went beyond reducing subjective experiences of discomfort. Not only did those who receive fake ultrasound experience a reduction in pain, but the researchers also found evidence of a significant reduction of spasms of the jaw muscles and a significant reduction in swelling.

A further demonstration of the analgesic properties of placebo comes from a study by Fabrizio Benedetti and his colleagues. This study attempted to compare placebo response with the effect of the powerful painkiller buprenorphine. This study also included a no-treatment group. Benedetti and his colleagues studied fifty-seven lung-cancer patients who underwent a painful operation involving the surgical opening of the chest cavity to remove part of a diseased lung. Following the surgery, each patient was given injections of buprenorphine at half-hour intervals until the pain was controlled. Then, one day later, after the pain had returned to a high level, some of the patients were injected with the drug; others who were told they were getting buprenorphine actually received saline; and the rest were given no treatment at all. (The ethics of such studies can be troubling.) Those receiving the saline injections experienced a significant decrease in pain over the next hour, roughly equivalent to that produced by the drug, whereas the pain level of those who received no treatment increased.[20]

A study of the effects of name branding of pills to treat headache demonstrates a similar placebo effect. The sample included more than eight hundred women who suffered from recurrent headaches.[21] Subjects received prescriptions of pills with the instruction to take two tablets for any headache they experienced during the next two weeks and, within one hour, to record how much relief the medication provided. Half the women were given placebos. Half the placebos and half the active pills were physically identical to a well-known brand of painkiller, and labeled as such, while the remaining placebos and active pills were simply labeled as analgesic tablets. This technique in effect allowed the researchers to compare results across four groups of subjects: two placebo groups and two nonplacebo groups. By comparing the pain relief across all four groups, they were able to isolate the effects of branding on the treatment of headaches. In both the placebo and nonplacebo groups, subjects reported greater pain relief when they took the branded tablets. The research points to the power of authority in mechanisms of pain relief; more relevant for my purposes, it also supports the idea that placebos can have genuine analgesic properties.

We may not conclude from these pain studies, of course, that the placebo response reverses underlying pathology. In the studies I described earlier of sham surgery on patients with angina, for example, the subjects reported feeling better and having significantly less pain (in our terminology, *symptoms* of the underlying illness), but they did not get better (clinical *signs* of the underlying illness remained).

MECHANISMS OF THE PLACEBO EFFECT

We know that for a placebo to have an effect, it is not enough for patients merely to be given the treatment: they must be aware of receiving it.[22] This finding emerged from studies by Benedetti and others showing that when placebos are given to people secretly, so that they have no idea they are getting treatment, they report no relief from pain. Only those who are told they are being given a medication that promises relief will in fact report feeling better.[23] It is not the placebo per se that reduces pain: it is the promise of its effectiveness that matters.[24] R. Barker Bausell not only has found that the effectiveness of a placebo depends on the form and frequency of administration, but he also cites studies showing that the intensity of a person's desire for pain relief contributes to the magnitude of the placebo effect.[25]

If the placebo effect requires the involvement of the conscious mind, does this mean that it is nothing more than a figment of our imagination, something that is all in our heads? Growing evidence shows that there is more to the mechanism of placebo than mere imagination; physiologically, the placebo effect is real.

In 2001 a team of researchers headed by Antonella Pollo published a study that sheds an important new light on the phenomenon of placebo analgesia.[26] The study design is complicated; here is Bausell's description.

> Following recovery from anesthesia, everyone in this study was given an additional analgesic, and then an IV containing nothing but a saline (placebo) solution was begun and continued for three days. The patients were then randomly assigned to one of three groups that were identical except for what they were told about their 'useless' IV: group 1 was told nothing at all about what was in the IV or what it was for, group 2 was told that the IV might be either a real

analgesic or a placebo, and group 3 was told that the placebo infusion was really a powerful painkiller. Patients in all three groups were then allowed to request anesthesia as needed and were given it when they so requested. . . . Over the course of the next three days, group 3 (the patients who thought their IV contained a powerful painkiller) required 34 percent less analgesia than group 1 (the patients who weren't told anything about the IV) and 16 percent less than group 2 (the patients who were unsure whether their IV was a placebo or a real painkiller).[27]

This study supports three important conclusions: the placebo effect appears to be real; it is capable of producing at least a temporary reduction of pain; and it occurs only in those who have been led to believe in the efficacy of the intervention.[28]

But exactly how does belief in a medication's efficacy translate into relief from pain? What is the mechanism by which expectations alone alleviate bodily distress? Is there evidence of a biochemical or other physiological basis for the placebo effect?

Classical Conditioning

One of the first laboratory experiments to study the mechanism of the placebo effect was published in 1999 by the noted pain researcher Donald Price and his colleagues.[29] Subjects were told that they would be participating in a study of a new topical anesthetic, trivaricane (the name also used for the placebo in Kirsch and Weixel's study). Price and his colleagues explained to subjects that in past tests the drug had shown promise and that their experiment was aimed at testing its analgesic effects further. In this study, the same inert concoction that Kirsch and Weixel had used was placed in two medicine bottles labeled "Trivaricane-A" and "Trivaricane-B." A third bottle contained only water and was simply labeled "C."

The first step of the experiment was to assess all subjects to determine their actual pain threshold by using a device that administered heat to the forearm. Once this threshold was established, each subject's forearm was marked with a label (A, B, or C) using ordinary Band-Aids. (Ever cautious, the researchers even varied the location of the label on the arm at random.) Investigators told subjects that the liquid in bottle C was a control wetting solution, and that bottles A and B contained different strengths of the analgesic being tested. In effect, the experimenters created three experimental treatments—a strong placebo, a weak placebo, and no placebo.

The thermal device was then activated, but the experimenters clandestinely adjusted the degree of heat administered to subjects' forearms to make the heat levels correspond to what the subjects had been told about the strength of the sham analgesic they had been given. In other words, the heat was turned down low when the device was applied to the area marked "A," turned up a notch when it was applied to the area marked "B," and tuned to its highest setting when applied to the area marked "C."

None of the medications had any biochemical pain-relieving capabilities at all, but the participants did not know this. Once the experimenters were sure that participants believed in the effectiveness of the fake medications (that is, they had come to expect maximum relief from the strong placebo and little or none from the other two), they progressed to the next phase of the experiment. It was explained to subjects that additional heat would be applied to each of the treated areas. This time around, however, the experimenters administered exactly the same amount of heat (the highest setting on the device) at the site where each medication had been applied and asked subjects to rate the amount of pain they experienced. Subjects reported gaining the most pain relief at the forearm sites to which the "strongest" placebo had been applied, the second greatest amount of relief to the site where the weaker placebo had been applied, and the least amount of relief from the no-placebo site. In other words, the reported pain differences in the second phase were due exclusively to the participants' expectations about the effectiveness of the different analgesics.

This study points to one of the processes involved in producing placebo analgesia: conditioning through the manipulation of belief, perhaps best known from the famous experiments of the Russian psychologist Ivan Pavlov involving the conditioning of dogs. Pavlov showed that when he paired the feeding of his dogs with the ringing of a bell, over time the bell sound alone was enough to trigger the salivation that normally occurs when dogs are given food. Price and his colleagues uncovered evidence of the same physiological mechanism at work in the placebo effect.[30]

Poppy Fields of the Mind

Though Price's experiment clarifies one of the mechanisms by which placebo analgesia occurs, it does not tell us what happens inside our bodies to explain how placebo-induced relief from pain actually comes about. Some answers are provided by research from a different realm of scientific inquiry pertaining to the discovery of a number of defensive chemical substances in our bodies that help dampen pain.

For some time, molecular biologists have studied receptors in the brain for opioids such as heroin, codeine, Demerol (meperidine), and the like. They have discovered that the brain has receptors for these substances, described by one scientist as "keyholes" or "satellite dishes" that detect and respond to the drugs when they have been introduced into the body.[31] Subsequent studies of these receptors led to the discovery that the brain manufactures its own version of morphine in the form of endorphins, which is shorthand for "endogenous morphines." A number of related chemicals have been discovered, known variously as endorphins, catecholamines, cortisol, and adrenaline. Norman Cousins refers to them as the body's "internal apothecary"; I prefer Bausell's term, "the poppy fields of the mind."[32] Physiologists now know where in the body they are released (in the so-called hypothalamic-pituitary-adrenal axis), what triggers them (pain, fear of a perceived threat, prolonged exertion, and strong emotions), and the chemistry of what happens following their activation.

Another set of studies strengthen the conclusion that placebo analgesia is real. They show that it is possible to pharmacologically block the pain-numbing effects of endorphins. Researchers found they could do this by administering the well-known opioid antagonist naloxone. The drug was developed to counteract the effects of opiates, but further clinical research found that it also blocked the pain-suppressing effects of endorphins, catecholamines, cortisol, and adrenaline. The researchers (Levine and colleagues) asked what effect, if any, naloxone might have on placebo-induced analgesia. If the drug negated the analgesic effects of a placebo, this would constitute prima facie evidence that the effects of a placebo on pain were physiological, not merely imagined. To explore this question, they administered a placebo medication to patients with postoperative pain and found the expected decrease in pain.[33] They then injected the patients with naloxone and discovered that patients who had experienced relief from pain when given a placebo now reported increased pain. In other words, administration of a placebo triggered some kind of biochemical response that was neutralized by the naloxone. The study thus demonstrated the existence of a biochemical basis for placebo analgesia.

In this experiment, Levine and his colleagues also discovered that the mechanism for placebo analgesia was the brain's manufacture of endorphins in response to belief and that the drug naloxone was blocking the placebo response in exactly the same way that it blocked the effects of morphine—by blocking endorphin receptors in the brain. Thus endorphins and other analgesic substances that the body produces naturally were identified as significant factors in the mechanism by which placebos reduced pain.

A further study in support of this view appeared in a 2001 issue of the journal *Pain*. Its authors administered naloxone to a group of subjects who had experienced relief from pain through a placebo. In this study, treatments were administered to six different groups of subjects to test the effects of placebo analgesia and of the opioid blocker on it.[34] Because of its complexity, the details of this study are not easy to explain, but Bausell provides an admirable and highly accessible summary.[35]

As in the study by the Levine and colleagues, subjects were given an inert substance described as a painkiller, and then the opioid blocker was administered to see if it interfered with placebo-induced analgesia. The study confirmed that naloxone blocked the analgesic chemicals the body naturally produced in response to the expectation of relief. The experiment thus confirmed the role of the body's natural production of opioids in the placebo effect.

What is true for the placebo effect also applies to its opposite, the nocebo effect—that is, an expectation of a negative outcome (such as increased pain) that is followed by reported negative effects.[36] Jeanne Erdmann explains: "Research has shown that nocebo negative effect is due to activation of a molecule involved in anticipation of anxiety termed cholecystokinin. Recent work on nocebo and pain by neuroscientist Jon-Kar Zubieta traced the nocebo effect to the same brain networks responsible for the placebo effect and showed that nocebo worked in opposite ways, to worsen pain rather than relieve it."[37]

Brain Imaging Studies of Pain Analgesia

Further clues to understanding how the expectation of relief may result in analgesic effects have appeared in several recent brain-imaging studies. In one study, subjects were told that the researchers were testing the analgesic properties of a new type of painkiller, an ointment that could be rubbed on the skin. In phase 1 of the study, before the ointment was applied, subjects were exposed to mild electric shocks administered to the arm and asked to rate their discomfort level. In phase 2 the researchers applied an inert ointment to the arm, telling subjects that it would reduce their level of discomfort. In both phases of the study, the brain activity of the subjects was monitored by fMRI scans. In phase 1, known pain receptors in the brain were activated when the electric shock was administered. In phase 2, the researchers found that these brain regions were inactive, and instead those regions responsible for instigating the manufacture of endorphins became active.[38]

The science writer Lauran Neergaard of the Associated Press describes another similar study, this one done by University of Michigan scientists who isolated the same phenomenon. The Michigan scientists injected the jaws of healthy young men with salt water to cause painful pressure, while fMRI scans measured the effect in their brains. During one scan, the men were told they were receiving a pain reliever, which was actually a placebo. Their brains immediately released more endorphins (which act as natural painkillers by blocking the transmission of pain signals between nerve cells), and the men reported that they felt better. One of the coauthors of this study, Christian Stohler of the University of Maryland, concludes: "Our brain really is on drugs when we get a placebo."[39]

The findings of these research studies of placebo analgesia point to a single compelling conclusion, summarized by Bausell: "We now have a bio-chemical mechanism to explain how the placebo effect is able to manifest itself. That mechanism is none other than the body's own poppy field—that is, its ability to produce opioids."[40]

OTHER FINDINGS FROM PLACEBO RESEARCH

The placebo studies most directly relevant to understanding reports of miracles by saints are those pertaining to analgesia. But others are worth considering as well. One set of findings suggests that placebos can help reduce inflammation. In the ultrasound study I cited earlier, administration of a placebo reduced postoperative swelling. Moreover, in one phase of this experiment, patients who reported experiencing relief from pain as a result of receiving sham ultrasound treatments were then given naloxone, the endorphin blocker. Not only did the pain recur, but renewed swelling occurred as well.[41] Though the precise mechanisms linking placebos to reduced inflammation remain to be uncovered, the effect seems beyond dispute.

There is also evidence showing that placebos can improve the healing of stomach ulcers. Daniel Moerman conducted a meta-analysis of seventy-one controlled trials of drugs treating stomach ulcers. These studies all had the flaw that they did not include no-treatment groups. For this reason, none of them considered in isolation provides direct evidence of a placebo response. However, by aggregating and reanalyzing their results, Moerman identified a pattern to their findings that provides strong presumptive evidence of a placebo effect. He compared all studies in which patients took two placebos a day to those in which patients took four. He found that in the first group, 33 percent were healed, whereas in the second, 38 percent were healed (a result confirmed by independent endoscopic examinations used in all the studies). The fact that taking more placebos results in greater improvement suggests that placebos can assist recovery.[42]

Finally, conditions such as depression and acute anxiety also appear to respond to placebos.[43] Though these findings come from studies that do not include no-treatment control groups, they offer persuasive evidence that patients' beliefs about psychiatric medications can influence their effectiveness. One study of forty-eight patients suffering from anxiety disorders divided subjects into three groups, all of which received a Valium-like antianxiety medication. One group received red pills, the second received yellow, and the third received green.[44] The colors were switched around week by week over three weeks, so that each group tried each color of tablet. Anxiety levels were reported by patients and monitored by doctors who were not told which color tablet the patient was receiving. The study found that color mattered: green tablets were more effective than yellow ones, and, among those who suffered from phobias, green tablets were twice as effective as red or yellow ones.

A study of depression provides further presumptive evidence that mental disorders are placebo-responsive.[45] The researchers compared patients being treated for depression with placebo medications in standard drug trials to those with similar symptoms who were on waiting lists. They found that those who were taking placebo drugs showed significantly greater improvement than those who were waiting to be treated. Adding credence to these findings are results of a brain-imaging study of patients suffering from major depression by a team of psychiatric researchers at UCLA, headed by Andrew Leuchter. The investigators showed that the brains of the placebo responders in their sample displayed changes in activity comparable to those of patients who had received antidepressant medications.[46]

Reviewing studies of placebo effects among people suffering from psychiatric disorders, Gary Evans concludes that although studies including proper no-treatment control groups remain to be done, the findings of existing studies support the provisional conclusion that "the less serious mental conditions such as anxiety disorders and most types of depression do appear to be placebo-responsive [but that] [w]hen it comes to schizophrenia, the jury is still out."[47]

CONCLUSION

We have traveled a long distance from medieval and early modern healing shrines to modern-day medical and psychological laboratories. It is now time to connect these disparate worlds by examining what placebo studies can tell us about the role of belief in appeals to saints for relief from illness. The most robust placebo effects involve analgesia, indicating that people who believe that saints can cure their illnesses might well experience immediate and in some cases even long-term relief from suffering. Such beliefs may also lead to the reduction of inflammation, recovery from stomach ulcers, and relief from anxiety and depression disorders. And in all of these cases, though there is little clinical evidence of placebo-induced cures of underlying conditions, patients who have been given placebos report that they feel better.

In explaining the faith in miracle cures during medieval and early modern times, the key question is not whether disease was truly cured by praying to saints, but rather what inferences, correct or otherwise, people drew from the empirical evidence that such appeals alleviated their pain and suffering. If the sufferers went on a pilgrimage, prayed to a saint, and in the end felt better for it, it does not matter whether the recovery was due to spontaneous remission or the natural course of illness. From the pilgrims' point of view, they took action, and it made them feel better; therefore they concluded that what they did had helped. From the perspective of the sufferer, the absence of a no-treatment group in a clinical study is largely beside the point. It is not what scientists conclude that matters; it is what patients conclude, correctly or not, about the cause of improvements in their condition.

The research reviewed in this chapter helps account for some of the miracle cures reported in conjunction with visits to healing shrines. Most conditions that medieval and early modern pilgrims presented to saints for cure were accompanied by physical discomfort. According to modern placebo research, the mere expectation of relief would diminish the activity of pain receptors in the brain and trigger the signal to the body to begin manufacturing naturally occurring painkillers in the form of endorphins. The relief pilgrims experienced came from the poppy fields of the mind.

The moral stigma that could arise from being ill, and the implications it carried for affected individuals and their communities, would have created a strong desire and hope for relief. Placebo research tells us these factors are powerful amplifiers of the analgesic effects associated with belief. In addition, the beliefs held by suffering pilgrims were shared and reinforced by those who were there to facilitate contact with heaven: the priests who served as spiritual brokers linking ordinary people to the saints.[48]

Finally, because placebos work only to the extent that patients believe they work, anything that enhances the credibility of a particular kind of treatment will help boost the placebo effect associated with it.[49] Herein lies the significance of the ambience of healing shrines. Features of the environment in which sham treatments are administered directly affect people's responses to treatment. At a shrine, efforts were (and are) made to convey the impression of a divine presence; powerful and nurturing authority figures reassured the patient that all would be well; caregivers offered support and encouragement; rituals lent gravitas to the proceedings; and public reports of miracle cures were met with acclaim. These features of healing shrines made such places ideal therapeutic communities.

The hypothesis about miracle healing that I advance here is my own. But I recently came upon a study by a team of neuroscientists in England that I believe supports it. The team is headed by Katja Wiech of the Department of Anaesthetics at Nuffield College, Oxford.[50] She and her colleagues provide evidence showing that religious belief actually alters the brain in ways that change a person's responses to physical discomfort. The study compared reactions to pain among a number of devout Catholics, who were asked to view either an image of the Virgin Mary or a nonreligious picture while electric shocks were administered to them. The religiously devout subjects were compared to a matched sample of avowed atheists and agnostics who viewed the same images. Using real-time MRI images of brain activity, the researchers established that pain relief for Catholics, but not for nonbelievers, was accompanied by increased activity in the right ventrolateral prefrontal cortex, which is the area associated with perceived control over pain. In other words, the image of the Virgin appears to have the same effect on the brain as does anticipation of relief: the areas where known pain receptors are located become inactive, and those that host the poppy fields of the mind become active.

The research cited in this chapter shows how belief in the perceived efficacy of the treatments we receive for our illnesses, and our faith in those to whom we turn for relief, can help alleviate our suffering. But the narrative does not end here. Other lines of research point to features of pilgrimage that not only powerfully affect how people experience their bodily symptoms but also actually induce physiological changes that can contribute to recovery from illness.

CHAPTER EIGHT

Framing, Confessing, Self-Efficacy, and Healing

For pilgrims, the actions they engage in before leaving, en route, and at the shrine are strictly means to an end, that of receiving a cure. But several lines of recently published research point to the intriguing possibility that such actions may themselves enhance the pilgrim's health and sense of well-being.

EFFECTS OF PLANNING ON THE IMMUNE SYSTEM

Earlier I recounted the words of advice given to prospective pilgrims by Richard Alkenton, to pay one's debts, set one's house in order, and "array" oneself. The need to plan carefully for pilgrimage seems obvious; less obvious, perhaps, is that planning itself may enhance the pilgrim's health. Recent research shows a relationship between what psychologists call "self-efficacy" and health.[1] Planning implies a particular state of mind, one in which people believe that by taking action they can effect change in their lives. Research by Albert Bandura and other cognitive psychologists shows self-efficacy to be a potent factor in choices people make about their work, education, health, and personal life. Our sense of self-efficacy helps determine the goals we set for ourselves, our commitment to pursuing these goals, our resilience in the face of adversity, the amount of stress we experience and our ability to tolerate it, and the level of accomplishment we realize.[2]

But it is the findings of studies of the effects of self-efficacy on health that are of greatest interest here. One of these is obvious. Self-efficacy works in concert with other factors to regulate lifestyle habits that directly affect our health. Research shows that if we believe we can deal effectively with sources of stress, we are less. bothered by them than if we feel we cannot control them. Studies show that exposure to the same stressors without the perceived or actual ability to control them can impair immune function. Epidemiological and other studies show that an actual or perceived lack of control over environmental stressors increases susceptibility to bacterial and viral infections, contributes to the development of physical disorders, and accelerates the progression of a disease. In addition, when we believe that we are unable to control adverse events, further complications ensue. Such beliefs cause us to distress ourselves further, and this distress in turn affects the immune system in ways that increase our susceptibility to illness. It appears that enhanced feelings of self-efficacy actually boost our immune system's ability to ward off infections and fight disease, and a diminished sense of self-efficacy increases our body's susceptibility to disease.

The relationship of self-efficacy to stress works in other ways as well. All of us are bombarded with taxing demands and stressors in our daily lives. If all stressors impaired our immune systems equally, we would become hopelessly vulnerable to infectious agents. But stress that is aroused while gaining a sense of mastery over adverse events actually strengthens components of the immune system, and the more rapid the growth of perceived coping efficacy, the greater the boost. Successful coping appears to result in a certain toughening of the immune system.[3]

This research points to an intriguing hypothesis. Enlivening pilgrims' sense of self-efficacy would strengthen their immune systems, thereby increasing the ability of their bodies to fight disease and infection. Because so many of the illnesses that were common among people living during the Middle Ages resulted from immune systems compromised by malnutrition, poor hygiene, and stress, the beneficial effect of an enhanced sense of self-efficacy, resulting from the decision to take to the road, merits serious consideration. Without the pilgrim's necessarily realizing it, the process recovery from illness might actually have begun before he ever left home.

AWARENESS AND INTERPRETATION
OF BODILY SYMPTOMS

Given the moralistic view that medieval people took of illness and the disdain and fear in which a community held its ailing members, sufferers must surely have longed for any sign of recovery. What effect might this desire have had on the interpretative lens through which pilgrims viewed their physical symptoms? Answers to this question are suggested in studies of a phenomenon that lies at the heart of the burgeoning field of health psychology: determinants of our perceptions and interpretations of bodily symptoms.

In considering bodily sensations that are associated with becoming ill or with recovery, it is easy to oversimplify matters. In the common-sense view, if we catch a cold and feel ill, we take steps to gain relief from our symptoms by applying well-known remedies, and we know intuitively from how we feel whether those remedies helped. Research on symptom perception, however, suggests that things are not nearly so simple.[4] In all but the most extreme cases, such as traumatic accidents, our awareness of bodily sensations can be highly variable. Moreover, the perceptual processes governing our efforts to understand what ails us, and to identify clues to recovery, are powerfully influenced by immediate context, culture, and past experience. Once we become aware of physical sensations and arrive at some idea about what causes them, our understandings are both greatly limiting and resistant to change. With illness, as with attempts to make sense out of other patterns and signs, we look for evidence that confirms our initial beliefs; we selectively exclude evidence that contradicts them and retrospectively reinterpret preexisting sensations to make our past experience consistent with our present assessment.

It is often said that seeing is believing. Research on symptom perception suggests that believing can also be seeing. It tells us that the commonsense ideas we hold about illness, regardless of source, largely determine whether we are even aware of bodily symptoms in the first place; once we are aware, they determine which bodily symptoms we attend to and which we tend to ignore; and for those we notice, these ideas dictate what, if anything, we do about them. The same factors that lead us to become sensitive to bodily sensations and their significance are also implicated in our assessments of whether we are recovering.

In an earlier section I described the findings of studies of hypertension.[5] The fact that hypertension is symptom-free gives considerable latitude to the beliefs sufferers hold about the nature of the condition. These varying beliefs affect the manner in which sufferers monitor bodily sensations. Those who think it is a cardiac disorder monitor sensations in the chest, take their pulse, become alert for irregular heart palpitations, and so forth. Those who attribute it to circulatory problems monitor their extremities for signs of discomfort or fatigue, and those who attribute it to emotional upset focus on mood states. Sensations consistent with their understanding of their condition are the ones they are most likely to notice; other symptoms, if any, are often ignored.

Important insights into exactly where we turn for clues to labeling and explaining our bodily symptoms are provided by a famous study published in 1962 by the social psychologists Stanley Schachter and Jerome Singer.[6] Their research showed that when individuals are physiologically aroused and have no ready explanation for the sensation, they label the state and describe their feelings by drawing on environmental and contextual clues. Moreover, once they have done so, other possible explanations for their feelings are foreclosed, and as more and more symptoms are subsumed under the hypothesis they embrace, their explanation of their feelings tends to solidify.

In this study, an injection was administered to the study subjects, with one randomly chosen group receiving epinephrine (adrenaline) and the other an inert saline solution. Adrenaline is a hormone (often referred to as the "flight or fight" hormone) released by the adrenal gland when danger threatens. When secreted into the bloodstream, it instantly prepares the body for action. Respiration rates increase, we perspire, our pupils dilate, the heart begins to pound, and heart rate increases. None of the subjects were told what they had been given. Subjects in both groups were then placed in one of two situations and asked to describe their feelings. In one, they were left alone; in the other, they were taken to a room with a person whom the subject was told was another study participant who had received the same injection. This person was in fact a confederate in the experiment who had been given no injection but who simulated a euphoric state. Schachter and Singer found that in the company of the euphoric confederate, the epinephrine-injected subjects identified their state of arousal as euphoria. In a second series of experiments, the confederate behaved angrily, and subjects also reported feeling anger. And, consistent with the researchers' theory about why this happened, once subjects had arrived at a working explanation of their feelings, they stopped casting about for alternative explanations.

In this study, the cues people drew on to interpret their own bodily sensations came from another person in the immediate environment. In the hypertension studies, people drew on commonsensical ideas from various sources. A study of medical students by the sociologist David Mechanic suggests another source of cues.[7] During their first year of medical school, fully 70 percent of the medical students he studied perceived in themselves symptoms of one or more of the illnesses they were learning about in their courses. The mere fact of learning the symptoms of various diseases caused them to compare what they were discovering through lectures and readings with their own bodily experiences. These perceptions were, no doubt, intensified by the fact that the students were sleep-deprived and under a good deal of stress, both factors capable of causing an array of noticeable symptoms. These physical sensations, which they might previously have ignored, were now experienced as salient and were interpreted in accordance with their newly acquired knowledge about disease.

Culture, too, has been shown to play an important role in the perception of symptoms and how we respond to them. The anthropologist Mark Zborowski studied how four different ethnic groups—Irish Americans, Italian Americans, American Jews, and those he referred to as "Yankees," or people of British descent—perceive, interpret, and act on bodily symptoms of pain.[8] He found that Irish Americans were more likely to seek medical attention for symptoms of any kind than were Italian Americans. Furthermore, for reasons that are not altogether clear, the symptoms for which the groups sought medical attention were different. People of Irish descent sought medical care mainly for eye, ear, nose, and throat complaints. Italian Americans were more responsive to symptoms in other parts of the body. The Jews in his sample were inclined to interpret pain as signifying an unspecified underlying danger, and they continued to worry about it long after it went away. The Yankees tended to respond to pain with denial, regarding it as benign and merely something to be endured. Irish Americans tended to be concerned about pain while it lasted, but then dismissed its significance and basically forgot about it.

Further studies indicate that the role culture plays in symptom perception may be far more consequential than we might suppose: it can actually affect patterns of morbidity among different segments of the population. Here the work of the sociologist David Phillips is especially striking.[9] In the Chinese astrological calendar, every year is associated with an animal sign; these signs repeat in a twelve-year cycle. In addition, years are associated with different physical elements: metal, water, wood, fire, and earth.[10] Some combinations of animal signs and elements are believed to be inauspicious: people born in those years are believed to be at greater risk of dying from certain kinds of diseases. Those born during "earth dog years" (an example would be 1898) are deemed vulnerable to developing diseases involving lumps, nodules, and tumors, whereas those born during "metal years" such as 1910 are susceptible to diseases of the lung. Phillips and his colleagues found that Chinese Americans (but not whites) died significantly earlier than expected (by 1.3 to 4.9 years) if they had a combination of disease and birth year predicted by this belief system. The intensity of the effect was correlated with the strength of commitment the subjects expressed to traditional Chinese culture.[11] For example, among the Chinese Americans whose deaths were attributed to lymphatic cancer (Phillips has data on 3,041 individuals), those born in "earth years" lived an average of 59.7 years; for those born in other years, the average age at death was 63.6 years, nearly four years longer. Among those who died of lung diseases such as bronchitis, emphysema, and asthma, those born in "metal years" had an average age at death of 66.9 years, whereas for those born in other years the average age at death was 71.9 years. Similar differences were found for other cancers, heart attacks, and certain other diseases. No such differences were evident in a large sample of white people who died of similar causes in the same period. The precise mechanisms that bring about these outcomes remain a mystery.

Framing

Our understanding of the roles of context and culture in an individual's understanding of bodily symptoms has been significantly advanced by theory and research on a process psychologists term *framing*. An essay that provides a broad overview of this research, by the social psychologists Shelley Taylor and Jennifer Crocker, explains that framing is fundamental to our efforts to make sense of our world, including how we feel physically.[12] Those who study framing speak about "schemas"—the rubrics, stereotypes, scripts, worldviews, and archetypes we use to try to organize and explain our perceptions. These focus our attention in ways that confirm our beliefs. In studies of illness, schemas play a powerful role in determining our assessments of how we are feeling physically, the ways we experience physical symptoms, and, based on these understandings, the actions we take with respect to them. As with the other studies I review, studies of framing show that once we arrive at a provisional hypothesis about the nature and cause of our bodily symptoms, we tend to selectively focus on information that confirms this hypothesis and discount information that runs counter to it. In consequence, competing hypotheses tend to be ruled out or disregarded. Once in place, the schemas we embrace lead us to engage in selective monitoring of other bodily sensations in search of further evidence consistent with the interpretative schema we have adopted.[13] And the evidence also shows that once we have formulated a hypothesis, our search for consistency generalizes to other sensations and becomes resistant to change, even in the face of disconfirming evidence.[14]

What is true of experiencing symptoms of sickness is equally true of searching for signs that we are becoming well.[15] When we are highly motivated to believe that we are getting better, we are likely to focus on bodily sensations and states that confirm improvement and, insofar as we can, to selectively disregard physical symptoms indicative of continuing illness. This tendency, of course, has obvious relevance for explaining why people who went on pilgrimage could become so certain that venerating saints had helped them.

Additional support for the hypotheses we have been examining comes from studies of pain conducted by the Harvard neurologist and pain expert Henry Beecher in 1946.[16] For many years Beecher had been treating people who had suffered major injuries in automobile and other accidents. During World War II he was assigned to work with wounded soldiers. He observed that the soldiers seemed to have a much greater tolerance for pain than the injured civilians he treated. He hypothesized that one difference between the two was that the military culture, like the culture of a contact sport, values and imbues people with a high tolerance for pain. He also speculated about what pain meant to the two different groups. For civilians, pain carried with it negative connotations involving loss of work, loss of income, disruption of daily routines, and so forth. For soldiers, pain meant removal from battle, providing an escape from an often terrifying, life-endangering situation. For one group, pain was unwelcome; for the other, it was welcome.

Beecher's observations spawned several other studies of the nature of pain, some of which I described in my discussion of placebo analgesia.[17] Pain experts now distinguish between the transmission of a noxious signal from the periphery of the body to the brain (nociception) and the overall physical, psychological, social, and cultural experience of pain.[18] Mood states (anxiety, anger, and depression, for example), focus of attention, context, and cultural expectation are all implicated in whether individuals report experiencing discomfort in response to experimentally induced nociception, and if so, how uncomfortable they say they are.

In identifying and responding to pain, the mental processes I have been describing can move either inductively, from bodily sensation to label, or deductively, from label to bodily sensation. In the Schachter and Singer study, the subjects perceived (artificially induced) physical sensations and labeled them in light of the behavior of the confederate. In the Mechanic study, the process worked in the other direction: students took the labels they had learned from their medical studies and applied them to their own bodily experience. The relevance of findings from both studies for understanding the significance of joining pilgrimage seems clear. For the ailing medieval pilgrim, the dominant schema would have been the desire to find signs of forgiveness for the sins that had caused the illness: namely, signs of recovery from illness. The supplicant would therefore focus more attention on bodily symptoms indicative of recovery than on symptoms suggesting continuation of the illness. There is no reason to think that by thinking in this way people would have gotten better, but it is easy to see how they became convinced that they were feeling better.

One additional factor is significant in our understanding and explanation of bodily sensations. Being ill and feeling desperate for a cure both entail a feeling of lack of control over one's life. There is a growing body of evidence that those who experience such feelings are especially prone to illusory patterns of perception. In a recent article in *Science*, the psychologists Jennifer Whitson and Adam Galinsky describe a series of laboratory experiments that confirm this hypothesis.[19] For example, those who felt a lack of control reported detecting nonexistent patterns in random noise, forming illusory correlations in information they were given, perceiving conspiracies when there were none, and resorting to superstitious practices to bring them good luck. Thus those venerating saints, many of whom would have been frightened by their illnesses and cast out of their communities, were primed perceptually to find evidence for what they most hoped to see.

The Meaning of Symptoms among the Miraculés *of Lourdes*

Though the issues are different, the studies of symptom perception I have reviewed apply equally well to the experiences of *miraculés* of Lourdes. Suzanne Kaufman observes that each of these individuals was confronted with two irreconcilable views of illness: her own, in which her symptoms were real, and that of the physician, who regarded the symptoms as imaginary and invented.[20] The longer this difference of opinion persisted, the more important it became for the women to maintain that they continued to suffer while under the physician's care. It was almost as if they felt obligated to continue experiencing suffering as proof that they and not their doctors were right.

The mythology surrounding healing at Lourdes contributed to a reframing of the sufferers' experience of illness in such a way that they no longer needed to cling to the idea that they were ill. It "freed" them, so to speak, to become well or at least to begin to experience themselves as recovering. Indeed, because of the religious meanings attached to long suffering and a return to health, this reframing in a sense required the women to present themselves as recovered or recovering, as added proof that their doctors had been wrong all along.[21]

Effects of Environment on Awareness of Bodily Symptoms

Framing is a mechanism that affects our perception and interpretation of bodily symptoms; another is related to the features of the external environment. The importance of this factor in determining our subjective experience of how we feel was first identified by the social psychologist James Pennebaker.[22] His interest in the topic began with his personal experience while exercising. Weather permitting, his customary daily workout was a five-mile run through the Virginia countryside where he lived. When the weather turned bad, he ran the same distance on a quarter-mile oval track. Pennebaker noticed that his times were much slower when he ran on the track and that he experienced fatigue more quickly. This struck him as odd, as the cross-country course was hilly and more challenging than running on the flat. It led him to wonder whether his performance might be affected by his awareness of the physical pain and exertion associated with jogging and whether his awareness in turn might have something to do with how stimulating, and therefore distracting, he found the external environment to be. He and a colleague, Jean Lightner, decided to put this supposition to the test.[23]

The two researchers hypothesized that the likelihood that we notice cues indicative of bodily symptoms is a function of the ratio of the quantity and salience of bodily information to the quantity and salience of external information.[24] In other words, the more stimulating and distracting we find our environment, the less likely we are to notice symptoms inside our bodies; and, conversely, the less stimulating our environs, the more aware we are of bodily symptoms.

To test this idea, Pennebaker and Lightner enlisted a dozen beginning joggers from an introductory psychology class and randomly assigned them to run one of two courses: an 1,800-meter cross-country course following trails through a wooded countryside or nine laps around a 200-meter track. Each runner was asked to run the assigned course on alternate days for two weeks. The researchers recorded the participants' heart rate and blood pressure before and after each running session and had them complete a questionnaire asking them about their awareness of bodily symptoms such as rapid heartbeat, shortness of breath, headache, and so on. Records were also kept of how long it took each runner to complete the course.

The results confirmed their hypothesis. Those who ran the cross-country course covered the distance more quickly, said they found it more interesting and less tedious, and were less aware of bodily symptoms. The more stimulating they found their external environment, the less notice they paid to how they were feeling.

Pennebaker and other colleagues have since tested this same basic idea in a variety of other ways.[25] Every study on this subject confirms the basic hypothesis that when the environment is not stimulating, people are far more likely to pay attention to bodily sensations and symptoms. And perhaps most interesting of all, one of the most important sources of distraction is other people.

These results suggest additional explanations for the healing effects of pilgrimage. Winter for medieval people was a time of intense tedium and inactivity, as the cold weather forced them to stay indoors for long periods. This meant idling away their time in dark, smelly, and cold rooms with little to occupy them and few opportunities for social contact outside the household. Pennebaker's research suggests that such low-stimulus environments would have led people to become sensitive to and overly focused on their bodily feelings. And there would have been plenty of physical symptoms, among them cold, hunger, insect bites, and skin eruptions.

On a springtime pilgrimage, then, people would have found themselves in a very much more stimulating, distracting environment, one encompassing the challenges of surviving on the open road, the stimulation provided by the company of others, and the break from routine. It is plausible that these conditions would lead pilgrims, like the subjects in Pennebaker's jogging studies, to become less aware of inner bodily sensations, thereby creating the impression that they were indeed getting better.

CONFESSING AND THE IMMUNE SYSTEM

However stimulating the journey, a pilgrimage was not simply a carefree holiday. Those who appealed to a saint for a miracle cure could not expect to receive it without first engaging in a serious effort to achieve a state of grace, which could be achieved only through the full and open confession of one's sins. Pennebaker has conducted another set of studies whose findings raise an intriguing possibility—that one side effect of the practice of confession may been a strengthening of pilgrims' immune systems.[26]

Confession, or the sacrament of penance, is a practice of the Catholic Church in which people may confess their sins to a priest (in a confidential setting) and receive absolution for them. The intent of this sacrament is to provide healing for the soul as well as to regain the grace of God that was lost by sin. These effects require full admission of the sins and an act of penance.

The experimental procedures described below are not precisely identical to the rite of confession, but they do share at least one feature that is significant here. "Opening up" does not entail a confession of wrongdoing or an appeal for forgiveness per se. But, like confession, it does enable an individual to express feelings and experiences that have been kept bottled up inside, often with accompanying feelings of guilt and anxiety.

Pennebaker found that when people who had experienced a trauma of some sort, usually psychological, were given the opportunity to talk about it openly and gain social acceptance for what had happened to them, the practice had dramatic physiological benefits. This study began with a finding from a study he and his colleagues had conducted on women suffering from bulimia. One of their most striking findings was that when a group of women who were bulimic were compared with a group who were not, the only major difference between them was that the women with bulimia were actively holding back a secret about a previous traumatic experience. They also found that women with other behavioral difficulties were far more likely to have had a traumatic sexual experience while young than those who did not. In addition, both groups—bulimic women and the sexually traumatized—were much less physically healthy than those who were harboring no major secret or had reported no early sexual trauma. His finding of a link between early sexual trauma and health was subsequently confirmed by results of a separate study conducted by *Psychology Today*, which showed that women who experienced sexual trauma in childhood had higher rates in adult life of ulcers, infections, heart problems, and illnesses in virtually every other category of health.[27]

Pennebaker speculated that it was probably not the trauma per se that explained these links but the fact that the women felt unable to talk about the trauma they had experienced.[28] They were burdened by a hidden stigma. This conclusion led him to hypothesize that those who experience any kind of a trauma they cannot talk about openly are more vulnerable to long-term health problems.

To explore this idea, Pennebaker conducted a second study, this one involving two hundred employees of a Dallas-based company.[29] He found that those with the most severe health problems had experienced at least one childhood trauma that they had not previously confided to anyone. Those who had been traumatized but never spoke about it were more likely to have been diagnosed with nearly every major and minor health problem about which the researchers asked, including cancer, high blood pressure, ulcers, flu, headaches, and even earaches. The nature of the trauma didn't seem to matter; the important thing was that it had never been talked about.

This led Pennebaker to design a third study, one of people whose spouses had recently died.[30] Here he compared those whose husbands or wives had died from accidents or natural causes with those who spouses had committed suicide. Because the suicide of a spouse is both painful and potentially stigmatizing, he predicted that spouses of suicide victims would be less likely to talk about the death and, in the year following the death, would have more health problems. Although this connection was not confirmed, Pennebaker did uncover another finding that was, in its own way, more interesting. The key factor was not how the spouse had died but whether the surviving spouse had talked with anyone about the death. Those who did were much healthier than those who did not. He writes: "Those who didn't talk about the death often obsessed or ruminated about it. . . . [P]eople who talked about their spouses' deaths tended not to think about the death as much as those who inhibited talking. . . . [R]uminating about the death was correlated with poor physical health. In other words, three factors were closely interrelated: Not talking about death, ruminating about it, and physical health problems during the year after the death."[31] Why this happened was not clear.

In Pennebaker's next study, he invited student volunteers to come to his laboratory and gave them instructions for writing about either a trauma they had experienced or a superficial topic. Of those who wrote about traumas, one-third were asked just to vent their feelings, another third wrote just about the facts without mention of their feelings, and a third wrote about both feelings and facts. With their permission, he also monitored their subsequent use of the student health service. Consistent with the results of his previous studies, he found that individuals who had written about their deepest thoughts and feelings regarding a traumatic event showed a significant decrease in illness visits to the student health service—a 50 percent drop.

In a final series of studies, Pennebaker joined forces with another researcher, Janice Kiecolt-Glaser. Together with her husband, Ronald Glaser, Kiecolt-Glaser had earlier reported finding that overwhelming experiences such as divorce, major exams in college, and even acute loneliness adversely affected the immune system.[32] Pennebaker and Kiecolt-Glaser now designed a study to see if writing about traumas could directly affect subjects' immune systems. Blood samples were drawn from the "trauma" group as well as from a control group of subjects who were asked to write about inconsequential matters over several weeks. Those who wrote candidly about trauma showed evidence of heightened immune system functioning compared with those who wrote only about superficial topics. The effect was most pronounced after the last day of writing, but it persisted six weeks after the study. Again, health-center visits for illness dropped for the students who wrote about their traumas.

By now, dozens of similar writing experiments have been conducted throughout the world. The subjects have included grade-school children, people in nursing homes, arthritis suffers, medical school students, maximum-security prisoners, new mothers, and victims of rape.[33] All confirm Pennebaker's basic finding that disclosing emotional upheavals improves the functioning of the immune system and therefore promotes physical health. It also improves mental health.

Pennebaker and other researchers have continued to investigate the physiological concomitants of disclosing inner secrets. For example, Don Fowles has found that the more people inhibited their behaviors, the sweatier their hands became, and the higher their skin conductance levels were (galvanic skin response is considered to be a robust measure of emotional arousal associated with inhibition).[34] Pennebaker's research shows that when subjects in his study were asked to talk about traumatic experiences in their lives, skin conductance dropped, and blood pressure, although it initially spiked when the subjects first talked about trauma, subsequently dropped below previous levels. He summarizes the results of this series of experiments: "When disclosing deeply personal experiences, there are immediate changes in brain-wave patterns, skin conductance levels, and overt behavioral correlates of the letting-go experience. After confessions, significant drops in blood pressure and heart rate, as well as improvements in immune function, occur. In the weeks and months afterwards, people's physical and psychological health is improved."[35]

Two other findings from Pennebaker's research are noteworthy. Among people who turned to regular prayer to cope with the death of a spouse, well-being was correlated with the frequency of prayer. It is possible that prayer provides an alternative medium for the practice of disclosing and confiding that his writing experiments had achieved.[36]

Pennebaker also discovered that, although disclosing benefits health more than not disclosing, there are special benefits associated with revealing inner traumas to listeners who are anonymous. The more anonymous and unique the setting, the more likely people are to make candid confessions.[37] This finding leads me to hypothesize that during medieval times, confessing to local village priests would not have had as many therapeutic benefits because it did not guarantee anonymity. Local priests were well-known to the individual and closely tied into networks of local gossip. By contrast, confessing one's sins to priests along the pilgrimage route, people the pilgrim did not know and would never meet again, would have maximized the health benefits of confessing.

Pennebaker summarizes the findings of his research this way: "Not talking or writing about upsetting experiences . . . can be unhealthy for several reasons. Holding back and not talking about an upsetting experience is bad in and of itself because of the physiological work of inhibition. . . . [W]hen individuals inhibit, they fail to translate their thoughts and feelings into language. Without resolving the traumas, they continue to live with them. The health benefits of writing or talking about the trauma, then, are two-fold. People reach an understanding of the events, and, once this is accomplished, they no longer need to inhibit their talking any further."[38]

Freud and Breuer

Readers who are conversant with the writings of Sigmund Freud and Josef Breuer on hysteria will be struck by the remarkable parallels between their ideas, Pennebaker's formulation, and the pilgrimage practices I have described.[39] Based on their clinical experience in treating patients with symptoms of hysteria (known today as conversion disorder), Freud and Breuer identify the physiological accompaniments of repressed trauma, explain how they can be eased through talking, and emphasize the importance of anonymous listeners. They state: "Each individual hysterical symptom immediately and permanently disappeared when we had succeeded in bringing clearly to light the memory of the event by which it. was provoked and by arousing its accompanying affect, and when the patient had described that event in the greatest possible detail and had put the affect into words."[40] Although in psychoanalysis the analyst is obviously not unknown to the patient, aspects of anonymity are retained: the analyst remains unseen, reveals nothing about herself, observes the rule of abstinence in communicating with the patient, and minimizes contact with and knowledge of the patient outside the treatment situation. Another theme in psychoanalytic literature is the importance of naming, framing, and describing events according to a coherent cognitive scheme, the same process underlying the studies I have cited about framing and interpreting bodily symptoms.

CONCLUSION

Beliefs and practices associated with pilgrimage could have had profound consequences for pilgrims' health. Some of the actions involved in planning and undertaking a pilgrimage might have directly strengthened the immune system and promoted signs of recovery from illness. In addition, the decision to journey to a saint's shrine, the reasons why people turned to saints for help, and the understandings they and others had about why they were ill could have decisively structured their perceptions of bodily sensations, including their judgments about whether they were feeling better.

CODA

I have explained the role I believe that social, cultural, situational, and psychological factors played in illnesses among medieval pilgrims. They suggest a narrative about how and why venerating saints and making pilgrimages to saints' shrines might have helped people feel better and even to get better.

HOW SAINTS HEAL

Imagine a peasant living in Western Europe in the thirteenth century who suffers from, say, serious difficulty seeing. She probably calls it blindness, but it is quite likely that her loss of vision is due to some other condition, most likely a dietary deficiency impairing night vision or perhaps conjunctivitis. Both conditions are usually self-limiting. Night blindness will resolve with adequate vitamin A in the diet, and conjunctivitis will clear up with good household and personal hygiene. But the term *self-limiting* obscures an important point: the condition will clear up only if the underlying causes are removed. So long as this peasant is exposed to the conditions causing her vision problems, in all likelihood they will persist, especially during the winter, when she lives indoors, continuously exposed to the pathogen causing the condition, and survives on a poor diet.

Neither the peasant nor those around her know anything of viruses or dietary deficiencies. If her condition is chronic, she and they will likely regard it as God's punishment for her sins. She knows that some saints are renowned for miraculously curing blindness; and so, if circumstances and resources allow, she will plan a journey to the shrine of one of these saints. By taking this decision, unbeknownst to her, she is already creating the conditions necessary to cure her disorder. Only centuries later will research by health psychologists, who label these actions as self-efficacy, show how the recovery might come about: her immune system will be strengthened as a result of her actions and initiatives. Her T-cell count will increase, enabling her body to fend off the organisms causing the conjunctivitis. When she sets out on pilgrimage, most likely in the springtime, the season will provide a more varied diet, including fresh vegetables, and so the night blindness will slowly begin to resolve itself.

Moreover, the journey may well alleviate our pilgrim's social difficulties. Blindness, like most other forms of illness, was deeply stigmatizing and exposed the sufferer to shame and ridicule, and so our peasant would probably have been shunned and isolated. By removing herself from the stresses and emotional turmoil caused by the judgments of others, she will feel the stress-induced burden of her condition begin to lighten. Hope and optimism will begin to supplant depression and despair, and this improvement in outlook may further strengthen her immune system. Instead of suffering rejection, she will now benefit from the social support of fellow travelers, not to mention the approval of family members and others at home. Her faith in the chosen saint's power to heal her (centuries later, health psychologists would describe this as a belief in the efficacy of the treatment) will create the expectation and hope of improvement and recovery. Without her realizing it, these attitudes will begin to activate "the poppy fields of the mind," the physiological processes that we now know to be effective in reducing physical discomfort. As she perceives signs of improvement, her faith and recovery will be mutually reinforcing. The benefits of a healthier environment, including exposure to sunshine and fresh air, will enhance

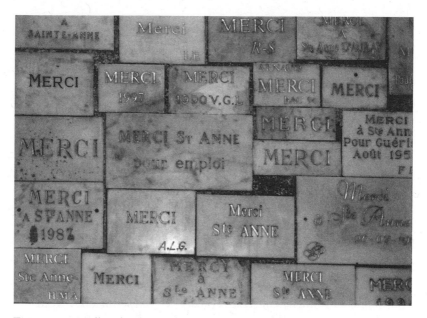

Figure 10.   Wall at the shrine to Saint Anne d'Auray in Brittany, where pilgrims have recorded their thanks for the blessings received, 2005. Photo by author.

these subjective impressions. The challenges and stimulation of travel will distract her attention from her physical complaints.

The rituals of pilgrimage will further promote perceived improvements in health. Unburdening herself, through acts of confession along the way, of feelings of guilt for various misdeeds will boost her immune system. By the time she reaches the shrine, all of these factors will have set the stage for a recovery in the form of a renewed sense of well-being and perhaps even a genuine cure. On arrival at the shrine, the excitement and satisfaction of reaching the destination and communal desire to find signs of the saint's efficacy will encourage further optimism and improvement; and partaking in any specific rites associated with the shrine, such as bathing her eyes with water from a healing pool, will intensify them. It is not difficult to understand how all of these elements could come together to convince the pilgrim that she had experienced a miracle cure. A similar script could be written for those suffering from many other common conditions, many of them accompanied by pain and inflammation. The credit for recovery, of course, would go to the saints. Modern research lends credence to the conclusion that people believed in the efficacy of pilgrimage for a very good reason: it seemed to work. They believed, and still believe, in the curative powers of saints less out of ignorance than on the basis of personal experience.

HOW OFTEN DO MIRACLE CURES HAPPEN?

How effective are appeals to the saints in producing relief or cures, compared with other measures one might take? This question cannot be satisfactorily answered without controlled, randomized comparative studies using objective standards for measuring improvement in health. Data from medieval and early modern healing shrines, including Lourdes, are insufficient for a retrospective study. But even from the limited and mostly anecdotal information available, we can draw some conclusions.

In part, conclusions about whether appealing to saints helps cure disease depend on what we mean by *cure*. Complete eradication of an underlying condition is rare; significant improvements in reported well-being are far more common.

The best available data come from Lourdes. Over the years, hundreds of thousands of sick people have made the journey to the famous grotto. One Catholic publication claims that between 1899 and 1999, 6,500 people reported to the official Lourdes Medical Bureau that they had experienced an immediate improvement in their health. Of these, 2,500 recoveries were classified by Lourdes physicians as "truly remarkable."[1] On further investigation, forty cases were ultimately declared miracles. (In the century and a half since the shrine was created, a total of sixty-six miracle cures have been declared.) Assuming these figures are roughly accurate, the odds of feeling better after a visit to Lourdes exceed those of winning the average state lottery; but if a major pharmaceutical company testing a new drug found that it benefited only 6,500 out of several tens of thousands of patients, and the illness actually went into remission in only 66 of those cases, the drug would probably not find its way to market.

It would be highly misleading, however, to compare recovery rates from the use of modern pharmaceuticals and medical treatments to those from miracle cures at medieval and early modern healing shrines. A more appropriate comparison is the effectiveness of miracle cures ascribed to saints stacked up against customary medical and folk remedies, such as cupping, bleeding, using leeches, vomits, inducing sweats, and drinking concoctions brewed from herbs and weeds. In this contest, the saints fare better. Appealing to them was probably at least as effective and certainly more pleasant (and less likely to cause additional harm). And the saints' treatments directly addressed the medieval understanding of the under-lying condition: the sufferer's moral failings, not what he ate, how he lived, or the germs or viruses he had unknowingly come in contact with.

Miracle cures are by definition exceedingly rare events, but this does not discourage the faithful from their conviction that they can happen. Perhaps this faith persists because of the critical importance of miracles to all visitors to a saint's shrine. For those who are ill, the incentives for belief are obvious. For others, including those visiting the shrine for purely spiritual reasons, miracle cures confirm that the divine is uniquely present and therefore available to them. As Goethe puts it in *Faust:* "The Dearest child of Faith is Miracle."[2]

MIRACLE CURES
AND THE MIND-BODY QUESTION

I end my analysis with two points, one looking to the past and the other to the future. A recent book, *The Cure Within* by Anne Harrington, explains the history of an issue that lies at the heart of my analysis—the mind-body connection. Harrington's aim is not to explain how saints heal, but rather to remind us that miracle cures are just one example of a phenomenon with a long history.[3]

She writes: "There is more to physical illness than can be seen just in the body; and more to healing than can be found in just pills and shots. Mind matters too: how one thinks, how one feels, what kind of personality or character one has or cultivates."[4] She shows us that this view of illness has been constant over time; what varies is how it is understood and explained, who explains it, and which groups and professions claim ownership of it. Her account of the mind-body problem is presented as a series of stories, each one resonating deeply with my own account of how saints heal. The chapter titles include "The Power of Suggestion"; "The Body That Speaks"; "The Power of Positive Thinking"; "The Effects of Modern Life on Health"; and "Ties That Heal." Each account culminates in an explanation of what modern-day biomedical, social, and behavioral-science research have to teach us about the episode.

The full details of the larger tale remain to be uncovered. I am confident that in time we will unravel the mystery of how mind and body interact, and we will understand when and how beliefs get under our skin and the role they play in illness and recovery. But wherever these investigations may lead us, one conclusion is already clear: belief, hope, motivation, and personal action are as important to illness and health as are any of the physical causes we are accustomed to naming. It is this truth that enables us to understand how it is that saints can heal.

VENERATING SAINTS ON THE INTERNET

My look toward the future considers the increasing role that technology is playing in the practice of venerating saints, especially apparitions of the Virgin Mary. Resources like the Internet and digital photography are transforming the ways in which people are exposed to and experience encounters with the Virgin. What do such developments mean for the possibilities of experiencing a miracle cure?

Paolo Apolito, an Italian anthropologist, studies and writes about Marian apparitions. His most recent book provides a compelling account of the ways in which worshippers of the Virgin now use electronic media to locate and experience apparitions. When he searched the Internet for the word *apparitions*, he was inundated with hits. (I did this recently and got 3,120,000 entries!) He reports: "One day in January 1998, Excite, one the best-known search engines, alerted me to the presence of 83,670 web pages; AltaVista, 48,030; Yahoo, 15,831; Virgilio, an Italian engine, 14,110."[5] Search for *Medjugorje* using Google, and more than one million entries appear. One website devoted to Medjugorje claims that it has received fifteen million hits since 1996. Apolito characterizes these findings as "a weird blend of . . . archaic elements with elements of late modernity . . . blends of religious visions and the Internet, weeping icons and television, stigmata oozing blood and high-tech laboratories, wheeling suns and digital video cameras, mysterious clouds and futuristic telescope-mounted cameras, divinations and faxes."[6]

These materials about Marian apparitions on the Internet offer much more than information about the Virgin; they are used by web surfers as a tool for the organization of Catholic visionary culture, a community where it is possible to join prayer groups and to participate in what amount to virtual pilgrimages and virtual encounters with the Virgin. For the faithful, the Internet is fast becoming the first source they turn to in their efforts to make contact with the Virgin, to look for evidence of her role in miracles, and to register their appeals for miracles. According to Apolito, for these users, the Internet is a place where "heaven can be seen directly, in which heaven speaks."[7]

This reliance on the Internet is having a revolutionary effect on the phenomenon of Marian apparitions and worship. So much material is available, in the form of accounts and photographs purporting to show evidence of her appearance, that her presence is becoming more and more commonplace. And because these followers gain the impression that she is omniscient, they are quick to spot her in all sorts of guises: not just in photographs of her face or entire person, but, Apolito explains, "In the form of images, shadows, silhouettes, lights . . . in windows, doors, glasses, bathrooms, parlors, bedrooms, shops, garages, soccer fields, streetlights, car dashboards, puddles . . . even plates of spaghetti, tortillas, buns, cakes, pastries, pizzas, pieces of fruit . . . rose petals, band aids."[8] Indeed, the Virgin is appearing to so many faithful in so many guises that Pope Benedict XVI has instructed Catholics who claim to have seen her to remain silent about their visions until a team of theologians, priests, and psychologists can investigate them. These inquiries will be conducted by the Congregation for the Doctrine of the Faith (formerly the Holy Office of the Inquisition) under new guidelines to be drawn up by a respected Spanish Jesuit archbishop, Luis Francisco Ladaria Ferrer. Claims announced publicly before investigation and clearance by the Congregation will automatically be dismissed as false.[9]

The images of the Virgin that appear on the Internet rely on photography to provide evidence of her presence. Pilgrims to sites where she has appeared in the past bring cameras and take innumerable snapshots in hopes that one of the images will include some hint of the Virgin's presence. (At some of these sites, the faithful are now advised to use Polaroid cameras so that there can be no suspicion of any Photoshop doctoring.) Less and less do those seeking evidence of the Virgin's presence kneel and pray; instead they point and click and, on the journey home, scrutinize their pictures. Those who believe their cameras have captured apparitions then post their pictures on the Internet.

In the past, Apolito notes, those who saw Marian apparitions were human beings; the new generation of visionaries consists of cameras. He writes: "It is no longer necessary to be good, humble, worshipful children, charismatics, saints, or whatever conditions traditionally typified the visionaries in the history of apparitions; all that is needed is to own a camera or, nowadays, to have access to the Internet."[10]

Apolito recounts one pilgrim's description of his alleged photograph of the Madonna while visiting Conyers, Georgia, a major site of Marian apparitions in the United States: "The image was shot with Kodak Gold 200, conditions were partly cloudy at the time with no direct sunlight. Unfortunately, I did not note the F stop of the camera at the time."[11] In place of details of pilgrims' devotions before and during their appeals to the Virgin, we now find talk of lighting conditions, lens sizes, and exposure times. Tests of veracity given to seers of the Virgin have been replaced by technical questions about the photographic equipment: "Did the camera function properly, or was there a malfunction? Was the film good or was it too old? Would a different type of camera or film have yielded clearer results? Was the lens adequate?"[12] To see the Virgin, perhaps all one really needs to do is purchase a continuously running video camera of the sort used for security purposes in the London Underground, set it up at a site where she has been known to visit, and wait. In earlier times, those to whom the Virgin appeared were viewed as people she had singled out, and it was she who picked the time and place at which to appear. Now even she becomes "an object, like any other, and she is not allowed to make the choice of invisibility."[13] And humans as receivers of these visions are all but obsolete.

These photographic materials, posted on websites, have made possible a new kind of pilgrimage (discouraged by the Church): the virtual pilgrimage. Computer users can now search the Internet for pictures of the Madonna and worship her image on their computer screens.[14] Click on such a site, and it will take you on a spiritual journey in the comfort of your own home. Apolito writes: "The exploration of Web sites . . . offers virtual stopovers and way stations, where physical movement is replaced by a shuttling from one link to another, with accompanying prayers and other ritual practices; . . . there is information and pictures of holy places and historical sites related to the apparition . . . you are invited to recite prayers or listen to sacred music with an image, the face of the Madonna or Jesus, or perhaps simply a legend reading: 'recite the Hail Mary.'"[15] And, like pilgrimages of the past, which were fraught with dangers, virtual pilgrimages carry spiritual risks. Google *Madonna* to find a website that invites you to join a virtual pilgrimage: if you follow the wrong links, you will quickly find yourself immersed in the world of pop music, or even in the lurid world of pornography.[16]

On a virtual pilgrimage, all of the rituals I have described as integral to the act of venerating the saint go by the board. Not surprisingly, so do miracle cures. According to Apolito, thus far there has never been a reported instance of a cure being granted to a virtual pilgrim appealing to the Virgin or another saint for relief from physical suffering, and my own search of the Internet for evidence has yielded none.[17] Perhaps it is too soon to tell, but I suspect none will occur. If the analysis of miraculous healing in this book is accurate, the replacement of the rituals and actions involved in direct appeals to saints, as exemplified by arduous journeys to healing shrines from Canterbury to Lourdes and beyond, with photographic images displayed on computer and television screens robs the process of its potential to heal. It is like climbing a virtual mountain instead of a real one.

ACCOUNTS OF MIRACLES
AT MEDIEVAL SHRINES

Though seldom useful in enabling us to diagnose pilgrims' medical conditions, accounts of miracles from medieval healing shrines are nonetheless of interest for what they can tell us about the symptoms pilgrims complained of. This appendix supplements chapter 5 by listing some of the miracles ascribed to the most famous English saints.

The eleventh-century bishop of Worcester Wulfstan (1008–95) was said to have performed miracles while he was still alive, including assisting in the cure of a woman who had undergone the "ordeal of the hot iron," a practice employed to test an accused person's assertions of innocence: the person's hands were burned by a hot iron and bandaged for three days. If they had healed in that time, the person was deemed innocent.[1] Wulfstan was also said to have helped a local beggar woman, crippled since birth, who was made whole, and a monk suffering from fever.[2] Wulfstan was apparently also able to curse: his chronicler mentions a tree that Wulfstan cursed because it stood in his path, whereupon it was said to have withered and died.[3]

Following his death there was a rash of tomb miracles that continued for well over a year, leading one observer to describe them as "growing in number until as many as fifteen or sixteen were reported in a single day."[4] In his *Life of Saint Wulfstan*, William of Malmesbury provides the most complete list of miracles ascribed to Wulfstan following his death. William writes: "The divine acceptance of his virtues bestowed on Wulfstan this grace: that after the manner of the ancient fathers he should excel at driving away diseases." William lists fifteen miracles ascribed to Wulfstan's influence with God. In addition to the cases mentioned above, they included cures for madness; "the King's evil," a term sometimes used to refer to leprosy; a "monstrous tumor"; blindness; the cure of a nun's malignant tumor; the relief of a man "sore vexed with pain in his bowel"; the healing of a woman suffering from "a sudden malady" which "seized not only on one member, but on every limb, and stiffened and knotted all her joints"; and the cure of a man "smitten" after he had struck a young boy.[5]

William's description of the cure of leprosy is particularly graphic. He says of the man that the disease "had gradually so poisoned all his bodily members that you could not rightly say he had a body, but went about with a living corpse. . . . [H]e was all running with foul matter; horrible to hear, for his speech was a kind of hoarse whining." One of the people Wulfstan cured while he was still alive, a woman named Segild, told William that she had had a vision in which God told her that she would be delivered by Bishop Wulfstan. Through friends, Wulfstan was persuaded to write a prayer for her. He wrote on a scroll: "May Jesus heal thee, Segild." When the scroll was placed on her body where the pain was most intense, it eased at once. Eventually she experienced a full recovery.[6]

Like Wulfstan, Edward the Confessor (1004–66) was reported to have performed miracles while he was still alive, and, as with Wulfstan, following Edward's death in 1066 the list of miracles ascribed to him quickly grew.[7] They included a hunchback cured at Edward's tomb; the restoration of sight to six blind men and a one-eyed man; a girl cured at the tomb; and a monk cured of quatran fever. Edward's biographer, Aelred, writes that the fever had troubled the man for six months, "for it seems to be the nature of the disease to be recurrent." His flesh was wasted, his blood weakened, his bones empty of marrow. He prayed to Edward, and then, according to Aelred, "at last when the Mass was over, he rose from prayer—and lo, all his pain departed and all his limbs recovered their original strength as if bathed by a fresh shower." Aelred also mentions a knight cured of the same disease and a monk cured from a threefold disease. He suffered from an abscessed wound that deprived him of the use of his arm, together with constricted breathing and swelling of the foot. After the monk prayed to Edward, the abscess burst; he then broke out in a sweat and could breathe, and the swelling in his foot subsided.[8]

The lists of miracles ascribed to other saints read very much the same way. Saint Edmund of Abingdon is said to have restored sight to the blind, cleansed the leper, and cured the paralyzed.[9] Hugh of Lincoln, while still living, reportedly cured cases of demonic possession, caused seizures and convulsions to cease, brought the dead back to life, healed the crippled, and cured those suffering from dropsy. The petition on behalf of his canonization mentions other miracles ascribed to him after he had died, including cures of "four cases of quinsy, one of 'fustula gutta,' three of paralysis, three cripples, two dumb men, two hunchbacks, one child restored to life, one case of jaundice, one man with pleurisy, the woman with the still-born children, four dropsical patients, the same number of blind men, and nine who were insane."[10]

Thirty-three miracles were ascribed to the eleventh-century Bishop of Sarum, Saint Osmund. His first and most famous miracle involved the healing of the fourteen-year-old Agnes, from Salisbury, described in my prologue. This event is recorded in a fifteenth-century document submitted by the dean and chapter of Salisbury Cathedral to the Roman Curia, appealing for Osmund's canonization. The list of his miracles also included the cure of a case of paralysis, restoration of sight to someone blinded by an injury, the cure of a young man who suffered a serious head injury while participating in a sporting event, and the cure of a man injured as a result of a road accident involving a horse. The petition also mentions another miracle that suggests the tendency of saints' proponents to exaggerate: the case of a pilgrim to Jerusalem who, some two hundred years earlier, had been inexplicably transported back to Salisbury in a single day in order to deliver a handwritten letter from the Virgin, personally addressed to Osmund![11]

NOTES

PROLOGUE

1. Daphne Stroud, "Miracles of St. Osmund," 108–11.

2. Ibid., 107–15.

3. Coffey, Davidson, and Dunn, *Miracles of Saint James*, 94–95.

4. John of Salisbury, *Policraticus*, writing about the shrine of Saint Thomas Becket at Canterbury Cathedral in December 1171.

5. Susanna Elm, "Captive Crowds," 133.

6. Quoted in Ruth Harris, *Lourdes*, 315.

7. See, for example, Joe Nickell, *Looking for a Miracle;* Ronald Finucane, *Miracles and Pilgrims*, 59–82; Jonathan Sumption, *The Age of Pilgrimage*, 111–21.

8. Robert Scott, *The Gothic Enterprise*.

9. Brian Fagan, *The Great Warming*, 3.

10. See Scott, *Gothic Enterprise*, 36–42; Brian Nilson, *Cathedral Shrines of Medieval England*, 134–43.

11. See Philip Ball, *Universe of Stone*, 271–72.

12. Nilson, *Cathedral Shrines*, 113.

13. Phillipp Schofield, *Peasant and Community in Medieval England, 1200–1500*, 7. Even lesser shrines drew large crowds for the times. To cite a single example, Nilson estimates that in the year 1335, some eight thousand visitors were attracted to the shrine of Saint Hugh at Lincoln Cathedral. For information about revenues derived from this and other shrines of medieval England, see Nilson, *Cathedral Shrines*, 114–17.

14. Edwin Abbott, *St. Thomas of Canterbury*, 227, 244.

15. Geoffrey Chaucer, *The Canterbury Tales*, 5.

16. See, for example, Finucane, *Miracles and Pilgrims*, 59–82; Sumption, *Age of Pilgrimage*, 111–21.

17. See, for example, Phil Cousineau, *The Art of Pilgrimage;* Robert Torrance, *The Spiritual Quest;* Joseph Campbell, *Pathways to Bliss;* Joseph Campbell and Bill Moyers, *The Power of Myth;* Victor Turner and Edith Turner, *Image and Pilgrimage in Christian Culture;* Lauren Artress, *Walking the Sacred Path;* and Bruce Chatwin's best-selling book *The Songlines.*

18. Scott, *Gothic Enterprise*, 203–8.

19. For an account of the historical roots of pilgrimage, see Elm, "Captive Crowds," 134, 137–40. For accounts of sacred travel in different cultures and religions, see Simon Coleman and John Elsner, *Pilgrimage:* on the classical world, 10–33; in Judaism, 34–51; in Islam, 42–73; in the Indian religions, 136–65; and in Christianity from medieval times to the present, 104–35.

20. Michael Wolfe, *One Thousand Roads to Mecca*, ix.

21. Ibid.

22. Ibid., xiii, xi.

23. See Coleman and Elsner, *Pilgrimage*, 136–66.

24. Elm, "Captive Crowds," 133.

25. Coleman and Elsner, *Pilgrimage*, 170–95.

26. For a fuller statement of the varied motives for joining a pilgrimage, see Eamon Duffy, *The Stripping of the Altars*, 44–77, 191; Cousineau, *Art of Pilgrimage.*

CHAPTER 1. LIFE IN THE MIDDLE AGES

1. Max Weber, *The Sociology of Religion*, 399.

2. Michael Goodich, *Violence and Miracle in the Fourteenth Century*, 2.

3. Recent experiments by social psychologists reveal the extent to which ordinary people still resort to magic and magical thinking to soothe the anxieties induced by uncertainties in their daily lives. For a report of this research, see Benedict Carey, "Do You Believe in Magic?" *New York Times*, January 23, 2007.

4. By *medieval* and *Middle Ages* I mean the period circa A.D. 500 to 1500. Many historians use the term *early modern period* to refer to the years 1500–1800. However, for convenience I use it more loosely, to cover the period 1500 to ca. 1900.

5. Hobbes was describing life in a state of war or state of nature "wherein men live without other security than what their own strength and their own invention shall furnish them withal" (*Leviathan*, 84).

6. For a general overview of peasant life, see Heinrich Fichtenau, *Living in the Tenth Century*, 333–45.

7. Phillipp Schofield, *Peasant and Community in Medieval England, 1200–1500*, 4, 9–76; Christopher Dyer, *Making a Living in the Middle Ages*, 155–69; Brian Fagan, *The Great Warming*, 3; Fichtenau, *Living in the Tenth Century*, 333–45; Schofield, *Peasant and Community*, 11–33.

8. Schofield, *Peasant and Community*.

9. Christopher Dyer, *Standards of Living in the Later Middle Ages*, 114; Schofield, *Peasant and Community*, 82–87; Josiah Cox Russell, *British Medieval Population*, 26–29.

10. Fagan, *Great Warming*, 5.

11. Dyer, *Standards of Living*, 114.

12. Fagan, *Great Warming*, 5–6.

13. *Hillsboro Free Press*, Marion, Kansas, June 15, 2005.

14. Fagan, *Great Warming*, 5–6.

15. Dyer, *Standards of Living*, 114.

16. Ibid., 119.

17. Carlo Cipolla, *Before the Industrial Revolution*, 23.

18. Ibid.

19. Malcolm Barber, *The Two Cities*, 12, 13, 7.

20. Edward Miller and John Hatcher, *Medieval England*, vii–viii.

21. Ibid., viii.

22. John Fuller, *The Day of St. Anthony's Fire*.

23. David Palliser, *The Cambridge Urban History of Britain*, 1:4.

24. Cipolla, *Before the Industrial Revolution*, 23.

25. Mark Kurlansky, *Salt*.

26. For a description of a typical seasonal cycle, see Fichtenau, *Living in the Tenth Century*, 333–58. See also Dyer, *Standards of Living*, 165, 168; Barbara Hanawalt, *The Ties That Bound*, 48–51; Cipolla, *Before the Industrial Revolution*, 90.

27. A. Roger Ekirch, *At Day's Close*, 27.

28. Emily Cockayne, *Hubbub*.

29. Dyer, *Standards of Living*, 191.

30. Ibid., 189. See also Cipolla, *Before the Industrial Revolution*, 112.

31. Ekirch, *At Day's Close*, 27–28.

32. Dyer, *Standards of Living*, 192.

33. Jonathan Sumption, *The Age of Pilgrimage*, 99.

34. See Miller and Hatcher, *Medieval England*, vii–x.

35. Schofield, *Peasant and Community*, 92.

36. Ibid., 93. See also E. A. Wrigley and R. S. Schofield, *The Population History of England*, 249–52.

37. Miller and Hatcher, *Medieval England*, viii.

38. See Shulamith Shahar, *Childhood in the Middle Ages*. She estimates that of one hundred newborns, on average half of them would die before reaching the age of five. See also Scott, *Gothic Enterprise*, 212; Cipolla, *Before the Industrial Revolution*, 127; Dyer, *Standards of Living*, 4–6; Russell, *British Medieval Population*, 173–74, and "Populations in Europe, 500–1500"; Keith Thomas, *Religion and the Decline of Magic*, 5–6; Ronald Finucane, *Miracles and Pilgrims*, 71–73; William Manchester, *A World Lit Only by Fire*, 54–56; and Hanawalt, *The Ties That Bound*, 45–63.

39. National Center for Health Statistics, *QuickStats*, April 15, 2005.

40. Shahar, *Childhood in the Middle Ages*, 146.

41. Carole Rawcliffe, *Medicine and Society in Later Medieval England*, 4.

42. J. D. Dawes and J. R. Magilton, "The Cemetery of St. Helen-on-the-Walls, Aldwark."

43. Hans-Werner Goetz, *Life in the Middle Ages*, 17.

44. Richard Holt, "Society and Population, 600–1300," 101.

45. Dawes and Magilton, "Cemetery of St. Helen-on-the-Walls."

46. Barbara Harvey, *Living and Dying in England*, 112–45, 236–38.

47. John Hatcher, "Mortality in the Fifteenth Century: Some New Evidence."

48. John Hatcher, "Monastic Mortality," 667–87.

49. Barbara Tuchman, *A Distant Mirror*, 95.

50. Roy Porter, *London*, 42.

51. Thomas, *Religion and the Decline of Magic*, 5–6.

52. Ekirch, *At Day's Close*, 23–28, 146; Hanawalt, *The Ties That Bound*, 27, 125, 145.

53. Sumption, *Age of Pilgrimage*, 99; Ekirch, *At Day's Close*, 124.

54. See Rawcliffe, *Medicine and Society*; Faye Getz, *Medicine in the Middle Ages*; Nancy Siraisi, *Medieval and Early Renaissance Medicine*; Darrel Amundsen, *Medicine, Society and Faith in the Ancient and Medieval Worlds*.

55. Cipolla, *Before the Industrial Revolution*, 127.

56. Ibid., 2–3.

57. William Chester Jordan, *Europe in the High Middle Ages*, 290–91.

58. John Kelly, *The Great Mortality*, 62.

59. Carlo Cipolla, *Miasmas and Disease*, 75.

60. See John Hatcher, *The Black Death*, 36, 135–36, 130, ix, 163–64.

61. The role of rats and fleas in the spread of the Black Death is now a matter of some debate. See Susan Scott and Christopher Duncan, *Return of the Black Death*.

62. Jordan, *Europe in the High Middle Ages*, 295; Cipolla, *Miasmas and Disease*, 3.

63. Jordan, *Europe in the High Middle Ages*, 296.

64. Carlo Cipolla, *Faith, Reason and the Plague*.

65. Ibid., 18, 23.

66. This action may well have been prompted by a papal declaration. A series of popes periodically instructed bishops to warn local parishioners of the true cause of the plague—sin—and to urge them to confess, pray, attend mass, and join processions. For an account of papal and English bishopric actions during the plague of 1348, see Hatcher, *Black Death*, xiv, 59–61. The problem of infection through physical contact with others was compounded by the insistence of religious figures that God would not permit the pestilence to invade places of worship. Ibid., 186.

67. Cipolla, *Faith, Reason and the Plague*, 42.

68. Hatcher, *Black Death*, 140–41, 166–78.

69. Ibid., 180, 208–46, 37 (quote), 145, 172–73, 176.

70. Centers for Disease Control, "Death Rates by Age and Age-Adjusted Death Rates for 15 Leading Causes of Death in 2006."

71. Hanawalt, *The Ties That Bound*, 183.

72. Rawcliffe, *Medicine and Society*, 4.

73. Ekirch, *At Day's Close*, 23–24.

74. Hanawalt, *The Ties That Bound*; Ekirch, *At Day's Close*, 25.

75. Ekirch, *At Day's Close*, 42; Manchester, *A World Lit Only by Fire*, 6.

76. Ekirch, *At Day's Close*, 95–97.

77. Ibid., 76.

78. Penny Roberts, "Agencies Human and Divine," 9–27; Ekirch, *At Day's Close*, 51–52.

79. Ekirch, *At Day's Close*, 49.

80. Peter Marshall, "Fear, Purgatory and Polemic in Reformation England," 150–66.

81. See William Naphy and Penny Roberts, *Fear in Early Modern Society*, for informative essays about these and other sources of fear in the medieval population.

82. Sumption, *Age of Pilgrimage*, 9–20.

83. Goodich, *Violence and Miracle*, 104, 110, 113, 23–24. See also Ekirch, *At Day's Close*, 9, 10.

84. Manchester, *A World Lit Only by Fire*, 6.

85. Will Coster, "Fear and Friction in Urban Communities during the English Civil War," 100–177.

86. Rawcliffe, *Medicine and Society*, 74.

87. Goodich, *Violence and Miracle*, 43.

88. Miller and Hatcher, *Medieval England*, 14.

89. J. R. Hale, "Violence in the Middle Ages: A Background."

90. Ekirch, *At Day's Close*, 45.

91. Fichtenau, *Living in the Tenth Century*, 141–44.

92. Evelyn Kitayama, "Culture and the Expression of Emotion," 5:3134–39.

93. J. Pitt-Rivers, "Honor and Social Status."

94. Richard Nisbett and Dov Cohen, *Culture of Honor.* See also L. Berkowitz, "Psychology of Aggression in Adulthood."

95. David Nirenberg, *Communities of Violence*, 18–40.

96. Raymond van Dam, *Saints and Their Miracles in Late Antique Gaul*, 82.

97. Fichtenau, *Living in the Tenth Century*, 309.

98. Rawcliffe, *Medicine and Society*, 32, 33.

99. Sumption, *Age of Pilgrimage*, 102–3.

100. Rawcliffe, *Medicine and Society*, 10, 58, 68, 67–70, 74, 10; see also Siraisi, *Medieval and Early Renaissance Medicine*, 115–52.

101. Rawcliffe, *Medicine and Society*, 68, 87.

102. Ibid., 88, 89.

103. Siraisi, *Medieval and Early Renaissance Medicine*, 120.

104. Getz, *Medicine in the Middle Ages*, 90.

105. Schofield, *Peasant and Community*, 5.

106. Dyer, *Making a Living*, 184–86.

107. Schofield, *Peasant and Community*, 6; Dyer, *Making a Living*, 185.

108. Schofield, *Peasant and Community*, 187.

109. Katherine French, "Parish Life," 325–51. On the role of local parish churches in confession and communion, see R. N. Swanson, *Religion and Devotion*, 26.

110. Schofield, *Peasant and Community*, 187.

111. Ibid., 194–201, 330–31.

112. Daniel Bornstein, "Living Christianity," 22; Schofield, *Peasant and Community*, 186–212.

113. William Christian, *Person and God in a Spanish Valley*, introduction and 11–12, 42, 99–101.

114. Émile Durkheim, *The Elementary Forms of Religious Life*, 419.

CHAPTER 2. SAINTS

1. Heinrich Fichtenau, *Living in the Tenth Century*, 309.
2. William Christian, *Apparitions in Late Medieval and Renaissance Spain*, 13.
3. See Daniel Bornstein, *Medieval Christianity*, 77.
4. Donald Attwater and Catherine Rachel John, *Penguin Dictionary of Saints*, 1.
5. Ibid., 4.
6. Peter Brown, *The Cult of Saints*, 5–6.
7. Attwater and John, *Penguin Dictionary of Saints*, 4.
8. Initially, canonization was informal, but over time the Roman Curia extended its control over the process. Beginning in the tenth century with Pope Alexander III, canonization became more complex and formalized, eventuating in the exhaustive processes that are followed today. See Robert Scott, *The Gothic Enterprise*, 203–8.
9. André Vauchez, *Sainthood in the Later Middle Ages*, 461.
10. Aron Gurevich, *Medieval Popular Culture*, 73.
11. Brown, *Cult of Saints*, 69.
12. Ibid., 1, 3.
13. Brown, *Cult of Saints*, 119, 50.
14. Patrick Geary, *Living with the Dead*, 77–92.
15. Brown, *Cult of Saints*, 50.
16. Gurevich, *Medieval Popular Culture*, 40, 17. See also Vauchez, *Sainthood*, 457.
17. Christian, *Apparitions*, 84. A novena is a devotion consisting of prayers on nine consecutive days asking for special graces.
18. Vauchez, *Sainthood*, 457.
19. Jonathan Sumption, *The Age of Pilgrimage*, 230.
20. Christian, *Apparitions*, 188–222.
21. Ibid., 15.
22. I know of no single registry listing the names of everyone, from earliest times, who has ever been canonized, but of one thing we can be sure: there have been many saints. The Roman Martyrology of 1584, referenced by Attwatter and John in the *Penguin Dictionary of Saints* (16), for example, contains

the names of some 4,500 saints, and they point out that that list is scarcely exhaustive.

23. Scott, *Gothic Enterprise*, 196. For additional details about the specialist saints, see Jacalyn Duffin, *Medical Miracles*, 40.

24. Duffin, *Medical Miracles*, 43.

25. Ronald Finucane, *Miracles and Pilgrims*, 39; Brown, *Cult of Saints*, 3.

26. Even on this count caution was required. Supplicants needed to ascertain that the date of a saint's feast day was accurate, lest the saint take offense at being honored on an incorrect date, much as we might feel hurt if friends and family celebrated our birthday on the wrong date.

27. Finucane, *Miracles and Pilgrims*, 33–34.

28. Gurevich, *Medieval Popular Culture*, 40.

29. Fichtenau, *Living in the Tenth Century*, 324–32.

30. Brown, *Cult of Saints*, 11; Bonnie Effros, "Death and Burial."

31. Achille Luchaire, *Social France at the Time of Philip Augustus*, cited in G. G. Coulton, *Five Centuries of Religion*, 3:28.

32. Geary, *Living with the Dead*, 32–33; idem, *Furta Sacra*, 34.

33. Émile Durkheim, *The Elementary Forms of Religious Life*, 99–126.

34. I am indebted to Chandra Mukerji for this insight and to members of the agency and object discussion group at the Center for Advanced Study in the Behavioral Sciences at Stanford during the 2008–9 academic year.

35. For extensions of this idea as it applies to the world of art, see David Freedberg, *The Power of Images*.

36. Vauchez, *Sainthood*, 36, 427, 428. Caroline Walker Bynum points out that relics raised an especially thorny theological question. Saints were considered to be immortal and their bodies glorious, not vile. But their relics were material objects, and like other material objects, subject to decay. One way to gloss over this problem was through claims such as incorruptibility and the odor of sanctity. "Holy Pieces: Attitudes towards Parts and Wholes in Late Medieval Devotion," lecture delivered at the Humanities Center, Stanford University, February 25, 2009.

37. Finucane, *Miracles and Pilgrims*, 26.

38. Sumption, *Age of Pilgrimage*, 24.

39. Gurevich, *Medieval Popular Culture*, 42.

40. Fichtenau, *Living in the Tenth Century*, 329.

41. Diana Webb, *Medieval European Pilgrimage*, 6.

42. Ibid.

43. See Gilles Fauconnier and Mark Turner, *The Way We Think*, and Gilles Fauconnier, "Conceptual Blending."

44. Anne Jacobson Schutte, *Aspiring Saints*, 73.

45. The ritual transfer of a saint's relics from one place to another is known as *translation*. Ben Nilson states that translations were among the greatest of all medieval ecclesiastical celebrations, accompanied by great ceremony and pageantry. Translations often were delayed for several decades after a figure had been canonized, to allow time to build an appropriate shrine and to raise the money required for the extravagant festival that was held in connection with the event. Nilson reports that these expenses could be in the range of one to two thousand pounds. For Thomas Becket's translation from his tomb in the basement to the corona built especially for him in Canterbury Cathedral, the archbishop gave two years' advance warning, to allow dignitaries and ordinary people to make arrangements to attend. The translation was celebrated with a banquet lasting four days and attended by 33,000 people. See Nilson, *Cathedral Shrines*, 6, 9, 13, 15–33.

46. Geary, *Furta Sacra*, xii–xiii, 14, 32–35, 44–45, 56–63, 65. Also see Scott, *Gothic Enterprise*, 164, 195.

47. Webb, *Medieval European Pilgrimage*, 8–9.

48. Gurevich, *Medieval Popular Culture*, 39.

49. See Nilson, *Cathedral Shrines*, 144–67.

50. Finucane, *Miracles and Pilgrims*, 113–42.

51. Ibid., 118–21. Also see G. I. Langmuir, "Thomas of Monmouth: Detector of Ritual Murder," 820–46.

52. See Scott, *Gothic Enterprise*, 203–8; Vauchez, *Sainthood*, 9–104; Michael Goodich, *Miracles and Wonders*, 69–86.

53. Vauchez, *Sainthood*, 81.

54. Nilson, *Cathedral Shrines*, 12–14.

55. These figures are from Catholic-Pages.com. Appropriately, within days of John Paul II's death, pilgrims flocked to a monument erected in his honor in his hometown of Wadowice, Poland, touching water that runs over its base and collecting it in bottles in the belief that it carried special powers of healing. All of this was reported in the context of a groundswell of enthusiasm to have the Church declare John Paul II a saint.

56. Suzanne Kaufman, *Consuming Visions*, 16–32.

57. Ruth Harris, *Lourdes*, 300.

58. Paolo Apolito, *The Internet and the Madonna*, 36, 22–78.

59. Gurevich, *Medieval Popular Culture*, 41.

CHAPTER 3. APPARITIONS

1. For an account of these and other such apparitions, see Sandra Zimdars-Swartz, *Encountering Mary*, 25–91.

2. Ibid., 94–95, 124–50, 232–37.

3. Paolo Apolito, *The Internet and the Madonna*, 6, 15.

4. Ruth Harris, *Lourdes*, 49, 72–80, 144; Zimdars-Swartz, *Encountering Mary*, 47.

5. Harris, *Lourdes*, 290.

6. Ibid., 288.

7. Ibid., 312. See also Suzanne Kaufmann, *Consuming Visions*, 2.

8. Given the commercialization of Lourdes by the Assumptionist Fathers, it is more than a little ironic that the official Church later condemned an Italian phone service of engaging in blasphemy by exploiting the faithful. The Church denounced the idea on the grounds that "for the Church a saint is . . . not someone to be commercially exploited." "Saints by Phone Service Condemned by Vatican," *Daily Telegraph*, June 12, 2007. See also Kaufman, *Consuming Visions*, 2; Harris, *Lourdes*, 288.

9. Kaufman, *Consuming Visions*, 16.

10. Zimdars-Swartz, *Encountering Mary*, 4.

11. André Vauchez, *Sainthood in the Later Middle Ages*, 147–56.

12. For one of the most detailed and impressive analyses of the social construction of a Marian apparition, see Paolo Apolito's *Apparitions of the Madonna at Oliveto Citra*. See also Peter Berger and Thomas Luckman, *The Social Construction of Reality*.

13. See Katrina Olds, "The 'False Chronicles' in Early Modern Spain."

14. William Christian, *Apparitions in Late Medieval and Renaissance Spain*, 213.

15. Ibid., 15.

16. Ibid.

17. Apolito, *Apparitions of the Madonna*.

18. Zimdars-Swartz, *Encountering Mary*, 25–91.

19. Ibid., 32.

20. Christian, *Apparitions*. Of the shrines Christian lists, ninety-five, or 52 percent, came to public awareness through intermediaries, 77 of whom were herders, 4 were plowmen, and 4 were hunters. In 62 of the 182 cases (34 percent) the sources of the apparitions were animals, who were reportedly able in some way to communicate their visions.

21. Ibid., 3–9.

22. Quoted in Zimdars-Swartz, *Encountering Mary*, 46.

23. Christian, *Apparitions*, 21, 217. In penitential processions, children were often placed first, as a way of putting the town's best foot forward.

24. Harris, *Lourdes*, 72–80, Zimdars-Swartz, *Encountering Mary*, 47.

25. Zimdars-Swartz, *Encountering Mary*, 27.

26. Harris, *Lourdes*, 3, 49, 144.

27. Zimdars-Swartz, *Encountering Mary*, 69, 72.

28. Ibid.

29. Ibid., 67–91, 12–16.

30. Margery Taylor, *Imaginary Companions*. Also see Paul Harris, *The Work of the Imagination*, 32–91; and Carol Nemeroff and Paul Rozin, "The Makings of the Magical Mind," 1–34.

31. Georg Simmel, "The Secret and the Secret Society," 332.

32. L. Lindstrom, "The Anthropology of Secrets," 13781, 13782.

33. B. L. Bellman, *The Language of Secrecy*.

34. Lindstrom, "Anthropology of Secrets," 13782.

35. Tanya Luhrmann, "The Magic of Secrecy," 161.

36. Zimdars-Swartz, *Encountering Mary*, 233–35.

37. Apolito, *The Internet and the Madonna*, 39.

38. Zimdars-Swartz, *Encountering Mary*, 241.

39. Ibid., 50, 62, 81, 128.

40. Ibid., 32, 85, 125, 128, 147.

41. Apolito, *The Internet and the Madonna*, 36, 15. For additional information about imitative apparitions associated with Lourdes, see Zimdars-Swartz, *Encountering Mary*, 59–66.

42. Christian, *Apparitions*, 20.

43. Ibid., 21.

44. Christian, *Apparitions*, 4, 81.

45. Ibid., 80.

46. Ibid., 83.

CHAPTER 4. PILGRIMAGE AND SHRINES

1. Diana Webb, *Medieval European Pilgrimage*, 78; Jonathan Sumption, *The Age of Pilgrimage*, 369; Ronald Finucane, *Miracles and Pilgrims*, 171.

2. Sumption, *Age of Pilgrimage*, 371.

3. See Webb, *Medieval European Pilgrimage*, 44–77, for an excellent overview of the reasons for joining pilgrimage.

4. Raymond van Dam's study of the shrine of Gregory of Tours finds that fewer than one-fifth of the pilgrims who visited it came simply because of faith. See Van Dam, *Saints and Their Miracles in Late Antique Gaul*, 126.

5. Webb, *Medieval European Pilgrimage*, 49–50; Sumption, *Age of Pilgrimage*, 136–59. As penitential systems developed for the correction of sin among both clergy and laity, pilgrimages came to be imposed as penance for certain offenses. Penitents were required to bring back with them a certificate from the designated shrine to prove that the penance had been done. It also became possible to buy one's way out of a penitential pilgrimage or to hire a substitute, known as a stipendiary, to undertake the pilgrimage. These substitutes were frequently employed to carry out pilgrimages for which deceased persons had allotted funds.

6. Susanna Elm, "Captive Crowds," 148.

7. Webb, *Medieval European Pilgrimage*, 45.

8. Sumption, *Age of Pilgrimage*, 280–98, 372.

9. Ben Nilson, *Cathedral Shrines of Medieval England*, 110.

10. Finucane, *Miracles and Pilgrims*, 44; Nilson, *Cathedral Shrines*, 110.

11. Nilson, *Cathedral Shrines*, 115–17. Nilson reports that the minimum in pilgrims' gifts achieved by virtually all shrines operating during this period was £5 per year, suggesting at least 1,200 pilgrims a year, or 100 a month. The average annual income for shrines affiliated with England's cathedrals was £100, representing about 24,000 visitors a year. On pilgrimage to Walsingham, see also John Hatcher's fictional *Black Death*, xv, 66–80.

12. Nilson, *Cathedral Shrines*, 148.

13. One way to explain the value of a thirteenth-century penny is in terms of daily wages. In my research on cathedral building, I learned that the average medieval hod carrier probably earned 2½ pence for a day's work; a gift of one penny thus represented 40 percent of his day's wage. The minimum wage in England today is £5.52 per hour, or about £44.16 a day, so the modern worker contributing a comparable sum at a shrine would leave a gift of about £18, or US$30.

14. See, for example, Finucane, *Miracles and Pilgrims*, 83; Sumption, *Age of Pilgrimage*, 103; Webb, *Medieval European Pilgrimage*, 59; and Van Dam, *Saints and Their Miracles*, 126.

15. Van Dam, *Saints and Their Miracles*, l, xx, 88, 87 (quote); also see Sumption, *Age of Pilgrimage*, 106.

16. John Eade and Michael Sallnow, *Contesting the Sacred*, 22.

17. Sumption, *Age of Pilgrimage*, 105–11.

18. Ibid., xx.

19. Ibid., 90.

20. Aron Gurevich, *Medieval Popular Culture*, 55.

21. Sumption, *Age of Pilgrimage*, 7.

22. Van Dam, *Saints and Their Miracles*, 6.

23. Ibid., 90. See also Harris, *Lourdes*, 294.

24. Eamon Duffy, *The Stripping of the Altars*, 189.

25. Suzanne Kaufman, *Consuming Visions*, 97, 126, 127; William Christian, *Apparitions in Late Medieval and Renaissance Spain*, 4.

26. Ruth Harris, *Lourdes*, 293.

27. Kaufman, *Consuming Visions*, 97.

28. The predominance of women as recipients of miracle cures is not limited to Lourdes. In her study of *positios* (bound testimonials of miracles) in the Vatican Library, Jacalyn Duffin reports that among miracles reported after the eighteenth century, there are nearly twice as many female *miraculées* as male. See Duffin, *Medical Miracles*, 52. See also Caroline Walker Bynum, "Bodily Miracles and the Resurrection of the Body."

29. Kaufman, *Consuming Visions*, 96–97.

30. Ibid., 96–97, 137, 144.

31. Ibid., 140.

32. Robert Orsi, "Thank You, St. Jude," quoted in ibid., 141, 142.

33. Harris, *Lourdes*, 305–6; Christian, *Apparitions*, 81–82.

34. Sumption, *Age of Pilgrimage*, 5–6.

35. Victor Turner and Edith Turner, *Image and Pilgrimage*, 4, 7.

36. Van Dam, *Saints and Their Miracles*, 102.

37. Peter Brown, *The Cult of Saints*, 113.

38. Ibid., 87.

39. Geoffrey Chaucer, *The Canterbury Tales*, 5.

40. Ben Nilson, *Cathedral Shrines*, 113–16; Finucane, *Miracles and Pilgrims*, 48.

41. Sumption, *Age of Pilgrimage*, 239. For additional details, see 239–44.

42. Webb, *Medieval European Pilgrimage*, 19.

43. See Sumption, *Age of Pilgrimage*, 428–39; Neil Smelser, *The Odyssey Experience*, 14, 53, 55.

44. Van Dam, *Saints and Their Miracles*, 117–35.

45. Webb, *Medieval European Pilgrimage*, 38–39.

46. William Melczer, *The Pilgrim's Guide to Santiago de Compostela*, 50, 45.

47. Ibid. Also see Sumption, *Age of Pilgrimage*, 253–55.

48. Raymond Van Dam, *Saints and Their Miracles*, 252.

49. Melczer, *Pilgrim's Guide*, 54.

50. Ibid., 47–49.

51. See Smelser, *Odyssey Experience*, 10–12, 52–53.

52. Turner and Turner, *Image and Pilgrimage*, 2; Brown, *Cult of the Saints*, 87. For an especially compelling account of the spiritual and psychological effects of pilgrimage, see Conrad Rudolph's personal account of his pilgrimage to Santiago de Compostela in 1996, *Pilgrimage to the End of the World*.

53. Smelser, *Odyssey Experience*, 55, 63–65.

54. Turner and Turner, *Image and Pilgrimage*, 9.

55. For an especially astute analysis of this aspect of pilgrimage, see Smelser, *Odyssey Experience*.

56. Turner and Turner, *Image and Pilgrimage*, 14.

57. Ibid., 15.

58. Sumption, *Age of Pilgrimage*, 243; Christian, *Apparitions*, 132; Harris, *Lourdes*, 291.

59. Sumption, *Age of Pilgrimage*, 8.

60. Ruth Cranston, *The Miracles of Lourdes*, 17.

61. For a description of the ambience of a medieval shrine, see Sumption, *Age of Pilgrimage*, 299–307. See also Smelser, *Odyssey Experience*, 63–65.

62. Turner and Turner, *Image and Pilgrimage*, 15.

63. Lauren Artress, *Walking a Sacred Path*, xxii. Artress was for some time a canon of Grace Cathedral in San Francisco. In 1991 she installed a labyrinth modeled after the one at Chartres outside Grace Cathedral's west front.

64. Ibid., 35–38.

65. Finucane, *Miracles and Pilgrims*, 164.

66. Ibid., 166–69.

67. Ibid., 152–72.

68. Ibid.

69. Nilson, *Cathedral Shrines*, 144–90.

70. Finucane, *Miracles and Pilgrims*, 160–61.

71. Conversation with John Hatcher, February 11, 2009.

72. Sumption, *Age of Pilgrimage*, 213.

73. Ibid., 388.

74. Nilson, *Cathedral Shrines*, 92.

75. Webb, *Medieval European Pilgrimage*, 65–66, 2; Turner and Turner, *Image and Pilgrimage*, 206–7.

76. Quoted in Erwin Panofsky, *Abbot Suger,* 89.

77. Sumption, *Age of Pilgrimage,* 111–13.

78. See Cranston, *Miracle of Lourdes,* 47–54, 94–103; Harris, *Lourdes,* 246–87.

79. Sumption, *Age of Pilgrimage,* 300.

80. Kaufman, *Consuming Visions,* 106.

81. See Eade and Sallnow, *Contesting the Sacred,* 51–76, for an excellent description of the helpers and caregivers at Lourdes.

82. Harris, *Lourdes,* 246–87, 306; Duffy, *Stripping of the Altars,* 198–99.

83. Harris, *Lourdes,* 305.

84. Cranston, *The Miracles of Lourdes,* 32.

85. William Christian, *Person and God in a Spanish Valley,* 101, xiii.

86. Eade and Sallnow, *Contesting the Sacred,* 24; Robert Frank, "Pilgrimage and Sacral Power," 31.

87. Duffy, *Stripping of the Altars,* 197.

88. Harris, *Lourdes,* 286–87.

89. Elm, "Captive Crowds," 148.

90. Kaufman, *Consuming Visions,* 129, 131, 139–40.

91. Ibid., 131.

92. Ibid., 148, 138.

93. Ibid., 127.

94. Ibid., 19.

95. Ibid., 100.

96. Harris, *Lourdes,* 244–48.

97. Kaufman, *Consuming Visions,* 27.

98. Ibid., 31.

99. Ibid., 35.

100. Ibid., 35, 60.

101. Ibid., 51.

102. Ibid., 68.

103. Ibid., 66–67.

104. Ibid., 78.

CHAPTER 5. DISEASE

1. The Historian Hayden White wisely reminds us: "One of the marks of a good professional historian is the consistency with which he reminds his readers of the purely provisional nature of his characterizations of events, agents and

agencies found in an always incomplete historical record." See White, "The Historical Text as Literary Artifact," 222.

2. Books by medical historians include Carole Rawcliffe, *Medicine and Society;* Faye Getz, *Medicine in the Middle Ages;* Nancy Siraisi, *Medieval and Early Renaissance Medicine;* Darrel Amundsen, *Medicine, Society and Faith in the Ancient and Medieval Worlds.* Works by medievalists include Michael Goodich, *Violence and Miracle in the Fourteenth Century;* William Chester Jordan, *The Great Famine;* John Kelly, *The Great Mortality;* Robert Gottfried, *The Black Death;* David Herlihy, *The Black Death and the Transformation of the West;* Colin Platt, *King Death;* Philip Zeigler, *The Black Death;* Alfons Labisch, "History of Medicine."

3. See Tommy Bengtsson, "Mortality: The Great Historical Decline," and James Riley, *Rising Life Expectancy;* as well as Christopher Dyer, *Standards of Living in the Later Middle Ages,* 4–6. See also Robert Scott, *The Gothic Enterprise,* 212; Josiah Cox Russell, *British Medieval Population,* 173–74, and "Populations in Europe, 500–1500"; Keith Thomas, *Religion and the Decline of Magic,* 5–6; Ronald Finucane, *Miracles and Pilgrims,* 71–73; William Manchester, *A World Lit Only by Fire,* 54–56; and Barbara Hanawalt, *The Ties That Bound,* 45–63.

4. Finucane, *Miracles and Pilgrims,* 71.

5. See Sandra L. Zimdars-Swartz, *Encountering Mary.*

6. On Becket, see Edwin Abbott, *St. Thomas of Canterbury;* Ben Nilson, *Cathedral Shrines of Medieval England,* 172, 184, 146–50, 116–23; Frank Barlow, *Thomas Becket,* 251–75. Barlow also provides a fuller bibliography of primary materials regarding miracles at Becket's shrine (318–21).

On Wulfstan: Emma Mason, *St. Wulfstan of Worcester, c. 1008–1095;* Reginald R. Darlington, ed., *The Vita Wulfstani of William of Malmesbury;* J. H. F. Piele, *William of Malmesbury's Life of Saint Wulfstan;* Finucane, *Miracles and Pilgrims,* 131, 169; Nilson, *Cathedral Shrines,* 26, 42, 113, 165.

On Edward: Aelred of Rievaulx, *The Life of St. Edward the Confessor,* 162–82.

On Cuthbert: Alan Thacker, "Lindisfarne and the Origins of the Cult of St. Cuthbert," 103–22; Victoria Tudor, "The Cult of St. Cuthbert in the 12th Century," 447–68; Nilson, *Cathedral Shrines,* 45, 95, 161–62, 181.

On William and Frideswide: Simon Yarrow, *Saints and Their Communities,* 122–89; Nilson, *Cathedral Shrines,* 16, 19, 23, 36, 63, 91, 156–58, 170–72.

On Osmund: W. J. Torrance, *The Life of St. Osmund;* A. R. Malden, *The Canonization of S. Osmund;* Daphne Stroud, "Miracles of St. Osmund"; Nilson, *Cathedral Shrines,* 102.

On Hugh: Herbert Thurston, *The Life of Saint Hugh of Lincoln*, 105. On Edmund: H. Lawrence, *The Life of St. Edmund by Matthew Paris;* Nilson, *Cathedral Shrines*, 27–28, 52.

On Gregory and Hilary: Raymond van Dam, *Saints and Their Miracles in Late Antique Gaul*, 28–40, 82–115, 116–49.

On the other saints, and shrines in general: Finucane, *Miracles and Pilgrims*, 11, 132; Nilson, *Cathedral Shrines*, 100, 125, 144–67; Yarrow, *Saints and Their Communities*, 169–89.

7. Abbott, *St. Thomas of Canterbury*, 244.

8. Ibid., 227, 249.

9. Barlow, *Thomas Becket*, 64–223.

10. Abbott, *St. Thomas of Canterbury*, 229.

11. Leon Eisenberg, "Disease and Illness."

12. See B. Knauper, "Symptom Awareness and Interpretation."

13. George Engel, "The Need for a New Medical Model." For additional discussions of the distinctions between these two terms, see Ronald Angel and Peggy A. Thoits, "The Impact of Culture on the Cognitive Structure of Illness"; D. Jennings, "The Confusion between Disease and Illness in Clinical Medicine"; Thomas Delbanco, "The Healing Roles of Doctor and Patient," 7–23, esp. 10, 14; and Michael Lerner, "Wounded Healers," 323–41, esp. 326.

14. See Getz, *Medicine in the English Middle Ages;* Rawcliffe, *Medicine and Society;* Siraisi, *Medieval and Early Renaissance Medicine;* Labisch, "History of Medicine."

15. See Carole Rawcliffe, *Leprosy in Medieval England.*

16. Finucane, *Miracles and Pilgrims*, 73.

17. Jonathan Sumption, *The Age of Pilgrimage*, 86.

18. Finucane, *Miracles and Pilgrims*, 73.

19. Abbott, *St. Thomas of Canterbury*, 249–50.

20. James Cragie Robinson, ed., *Materials for the History of Thomas Becket*, 137–98.

21. Ibid.

22. Abbott, *St. Thomas of Canterbury*, 233, 224.

23. Finucane categorizes the conditions reported in miracle accounts as follows: illnesses of an unspecified nature, including people who were bedridden, in some manner disabled, or said to be paralyzed; afflictions of specific organs or areas of the body, connoted by the use of such terms as *stone, flux, dysentery, fever, toothache, insomnia,* or *cough;* disorders resulting in impaired locomotion

involving the hands, fingers, the legs, the feet or the arms; *gutta* (gout), dropsy, and other conditions that suggest tissue swelling or edema; skin conditions such as open sores, localized swellings, tumors, ulcers, abscesses, fistula, quinsy, scrofula, and "leprosy"; blindness, which included other eye disorders; muteness and deafness (according to Finucane, quite rare); mental afflictions of various kinds, including what were described as cases of demonic possession, visitations by demons, or simple madness; and injuries due to accidents or acts of violence. See Finucane, *Miracles and Pilgrims*, 103–11.

24. Eleanora Gordon, "Child Health in the Middle Ages As Seen in the Miracles of Five English Saints, A.D. 1150–1220."

25. Ibid., 508.

26. Ibid., 512.

27. "Febrile Convulsions," WebMD.

28. "Encephalitis," WebMD.

29. Gordon, "Child Health," 511.

30. Ibid., 512; "Smallpox," WebMD.

31. One study that attempts to bring modern medical knowledge to bear on miracle cures in the Middle Ages is Jacalyn Duffin's *Medical Miracles*. In addition, Sumption cites a report issued by the British Medical Association listing six factors that can account for most miracle cures reported in modern times. See Sumption, *Age of Pilgrimage*, 120.

32. Finucane, *Miracles and Pilgrims*, 78; Sumption, *Age of Pilgrimage*, 114.

33. R. Barker Bausell, *Snake Oil Science*, 47–51.

34. Ibid., 48.

35. Riley, *Rising Life Expectancy*.

36. Sumption, *Age of Pilgrimage*, 112–13.

37. "Retinoids," WebMD.

38. Gary Evans, "Crowding and Other Environmental Stressors," 3018–22.

CHAPTER 6. THE ROLE OF STRESS IN ILLNESS

1. For overviews of research on this topic, see B. M. Kulielka and C. Kirschbaum, "Stress and Health Research"; M. Biondi, "Effects of Stress on Immune Functions."

2. Kulielka and Kirschbaum, "Stress and Health," 15173. A *risk factor* is a factor (such as heredity, diet, or environmental exposure to a chemical) that has

been shown to increase a person's chances of contracting a disease in a specified time period.

3. Ibid.; S. B. Manuck et al., "Studies of Psychosocial Influences on Coronary Artery Atherogenesis in Cynomolgus Monkeys"; Biondi, "Effects of Stress," 189–226.

4. Kulielka and Kirschbaum, "Stress and Health," 15171–72.

5. Ibid., 15172.

6. Greg Bishop, "Emotions and Health," 4455, 4456.

7. See C. Peterson, "Explanatory Style and Health."

8. Bishop, "Emotions and Health," 4455.

9. Ibid., 4457.

10. See James Pennebaker, *Opening Up;* I. Fawzy and N. Fawzy, "Psycho-educational Interventions and Health Outcomes." Also of note are studies showing that stress-reducing interventions can improve immune functioning in individuals with HIV. See Kulielka and Kirschbaum, "Stress and Health," 15173.

11. Sally Dickerson, Tara Gruenewald, and Margaret Kemeny, "When the Social Self Is Threatened," 1193–94, 1197–1209. (See pp. 1210–16 for a comprehensive bibliography of articles and books on this topic.) Cytokines are mediators of the immune response, a subset of which, the proinflammatory cytokines, initiate and maintain the inflammatory response. Inflammation is a coordinated bodily response to tissue injury or pathogen infection: it involves immune cells and their products entering the infected area, destroying the foreign organism or substance, and repairing injured tissue. Cortisol is a hormone produced by the hypothalamic-pituitary-adrenocortical axis. When this system is activated, cortisols from the adrenal cortex are released into the bloodstream, increasing blood pressure and altering blood chemistry.

12. See B. N. Henderson and A. Baum, "Behavioral Medicine"; K. Orth-Gomér, "Social Support and Health."

13. See L. K. Welin et al., "Prospective Study of Social Influences on Mortality."

14. S. D. Cohen, A. J. Tyrell, and A. P. Smith, "Psychosocial Stress and Susceptibility to the Common Cold." See also Henderson and Baum, "Behavioral Medicine," 1111–18; S. L. Syme, "Social Epidemiology," 4702; Orth-Gomér, "Social Support and Health."

15. K. Petrie, "Social Support and Recovery from Disease and Medical Procedures," 14458–61.

16. H. S. Gordon and G. E. Rosenthal, "Impact of Marital Status on Outcomes in Hospitalized Patients."

17. Gary Evans, "Crowding and Other Environmental Stressors."

CHAPTER 7. BELIEF, HOPE, AND HEALING

1. See Anne Harrington, *The Placebo Effect;* L. White, B. Tursky, and G. E. Schwartz, *Placebo;* Henry Guess, Linda Engel, Arthur Kleinman, and John Kusek, *The Science of the Placebo;* Eugene Brody, *The Placebo Response;* Dylan Evans, *Placebo,* 74; Daniel Moerman, *Meaning, Medicine and the "Placebo Effect";* Arthur Shapiro and Elaine Shapiro, *The Powerful Placebo;* Bill Moyers, *Healing and the Mind.* See also Richard Kradin, *The Placebo Response and the Power of Unconscious Healing.*

2. See Dylan Evans, *Placebo,* 25–43; R. de la Fuente-Fernandez et al., "Expectation and Dopamine Release"; F. Benedetti et al., "Placebo-Responsive Parkinson Patients Show Decreased Activity in Single Neurons of Subthalamic Nucleus," 587–88.

3. P. Iacono et al., "Placebo Effect in Cardiovascular Clinical Pharmacology."

4. For comprehensive reviews of this and related research see Evans, *Placebo;* Moerman, *Meaning, Medicine and the "Placebo Effect."*

5. Guy Montgomery and Irving Kirsch, "Mechanisms of Placebo Pain Reduction: An Empirical Investigation."

6. R. H. Gracely, R. Dubner, W. R. Deeter, and P. J. Wolskee, "Clinicians' Expectations Influence Placebo Analgesia."

7. R. Barker Bausell, *Snake Oil Science,* 135–36.

8. Moerman, *Meaning, Medicine and the "Placebo Effect,"* 66.

9. Ibid., 33–34.

10. A. J. Vickers, "Can Acupuncture Have Specific Effects on Health? A Systematic Review of Acupuncture Antiemesis Trials." Meta-analysis is a technique that examines multiple studies of the same topic to reveal findings and trends across the whole body of research. See R. L. Tweedie, "Meta-Analysis: Overview."

11. Classifying acupuncture as a sham treatment will no doubt raise the eyebrows of some readers. My rationale for doing so is based on Bausell's exhaustive analysis of carefully designed studies of the use of acupuncture to treat such conditions as acute stroke, asthma, Bell's palsy, headache, depression, elbow pain, epilepsy, irritable bowel syndrome, low back pain, neck disorders, nicotine

and cocaine withdrawal, shoulder pain, schizophrenia, and chemotherapy-induced nausea or vomiting. See Bausell, *Snake Oil Science*, 209–15.

12. Moerman, *Meaning, Medicine and the "Placebo Effect,"* 71.

13. Among the many reports of noteworthy placebo studies, see Margaret Talbot, "The Placebo Prescription"; Lewis Thomas, "On Warts"; B. Blackwell, S. S. Bloomfield, and C. R. Buncher, "Demonstration to Medical Students of Placebo Responses and Non-drug Factors"; R. E. Sallis and L. W. Buckalew, "Relations of Capsule Color and Perceived Potency"; A. D. Cataneo, P. E. Lucchelli, and G. Filippuci, "Sedative Effects of Placebo Treatment"; P. E. Lucchelli, A. D. Cattaneo, and J. Zattoni, "Effects of Capsule Colour and Order to Administration of Hypnotic Treatments"; J. P. Boissel et al., "Time Course of Long-Term Placebo Therapy Effects in Angina Pectoris"; Alia Crum and Ellen Langer, "Mind-Set Matters: Exercise and the Placebo Effect."

14. J. Bruce Moseley et al., "A Controlled Trial of Arthroscopic Surgery for Osteoarthritis of the Knee."

15. Gary Evans, *Placebo*, 4.

16. One survey found that fewer than 4 percent of clinical trials and meta-analyses published between 1986 and 1994 included both placebo and no-treatment groups. See E. Ernst and K. L. Resch, "Concept of True and Perceived Placebo Effects." As an aside, although it is correct that assessing the placebo effect accurately requires that one compare the experiences of the placebo group with those receiving no treatment, the same principle should be applied in assessing the experiences of the treatment group.

17. A. Hróbjartsson and P. Gøtzsche, "Is the Placebo Powerless? An Analysis of Clinical Trials Comparing Placebo with No Treatment"; A. Hróbjartsson and P. Gøtzsche, "Is the Placebo Powerless? Update of a Systematic Review of 52 New Randomized Trials Comparing Placebo with No Treatment."

18. Evans, *Placebo*, 28–34.

19. I. Hashish and W. Harvey, "Anti-inflammatory Effects of Ultrasound Therapy: Evidence for a Major Placebo Effect."

20. F. Benedetti et al., "The Specific Effects of Prior Opioid Exposure on Placebo Analgesia and Placebo Respiratory Depression."

21. A. Braithwaite and P. Cooper, "Analgesic Effects of Branding in Treatment of Headaches."

22. A helpful summary and explanation of some of the mechanisms involved in placebo response appears in Jeanne Erdmann and Bryan Christie, "Imagination Medicine." For an overview of research on this topic, see Kradin, *Placebo Response*, 101–68.

23. F. Benedetti, "The Opposite Effects of the Opiate Antagonist Naloxone and the Cholecystokinin Antagonist Proglumide on Placebo Analegsia"; Benedetti et al., "Specific Effects of Prior Opioid Exposure."

24. Moerman, *Meaning, Medicine and the "Placebo Effect,"* 106.

25. Bausell, *Snake Oil Science*, 136–37.

26. Antonella Pollo, Martina Amanzio, Anna Arslanian, Caterina Casadio, Giuliano Maggi, and Fabrizio Benedetti, "Response Expectancies in Placebo Analgesia and Their Clinical Relevance."

27. Bausell, *Snake Oil Science*, 139–40.

28. Ibid., 141.

29. D. D. Price et al., "An Analysis of Factors That Contribute to the Magnitude of Placebo Analgesia in an Experimental Paradigm."

30. Bausell, *Snake Oil Science*, 132–135. When patients are given medications (especially those with dangerous side effects, for which it is desirable to keep doses low) and the administration of the drug is paired with an extraneous stimulus—say, drinking sugar water—the subjects become conditioned to respond to the extraneous stimulus in the same way as to the dangerous medication. Thus it is possible to reduce the amount of medication given to the subject and still obtain the desired result simply by pairing the medication with the extraneous stimulus. See Robert Ader, *Psychoneuroimmunology.*

31. See Candace Pert, "The Chemical Communicators."

32. Norman Cousins, *Anatomy of an Illness*, 63; Bausell, *Snake Oil Science*, 153.

33. J. Levine, N. C. Gordon, and H. Fields, "The Mechanism of Placebo Analgesia." Also see Menchetti Sauro, "Endogenous Opiates and the Placebo Effect."

34. M. Amanzio, A. Pollo, G. Maggi, and F. Benedetti, "Response Variability in Placebo Analgesics."

35. Bausell, *Snake Oil Science*, 155–61.

36. Robert Hahn, "The Nocebo Phenomenon," 56. The nocebo effect can also refer to the power of spells or curses cast by people thought to have access to malevolent forces in the spirit world. If victims of such imprecations indeed believe that they are doomed to illness, misfortune, or even death, their beliefs may be self-fulfilling.

37. Jeanne Erdmann, "The Nocebo Effect."

38. T. D. Wager et al., "Placebo-Induced Changes in fMRI in the Anticipation and Experience of Pain."

39. Lauran Neergaard, "Expecting Pain Relief Triggers Real Thing."

40. Bausell, *Snake Oil Science*, 161

41. Evans, *Placebo*, 34, 58.

42. Moerman, "Cultural Variations in the Placebo Effect." This result has been replicated in another, more rigorous meta-analysis. See A. J. de Craen et al., "Placebo Effect in the Treatment of Duodenal Ulcer."

43. See Evans, *Placebo*, 36–42; I. Kirsch and G. Saperstein, "Listening to Prozac but Hearing Placebo"; Kradin, *Placebo Response*, 163–67.

44. K. Schapira et al., "Study on the Effects of Tablet Colour in the Treatment of Anxiety States."

45. Kirsch and Saperstein, "Listening to Prozac but Hearing Placebo."

46. A. Leuchter, I. A. Cook, E. A. White, M. L. Morgan, and M. Abrams, "Changes in Brain Function of Depressed Patients during Treatment with Placebo."

47. Evans, *Placebo*, 42.

48. Robert Scott, *The Gothic Enterprise*, 219–32.

49. Evans, *Placebo*, 200.

50. Katja Wiech et al., "An fMRI Measuring Analgesia Enhanced by Religion as a Belief System."

CHAPTER 8. FRAMING, CONFESSING, SELF-EFFICACY, AND HEALING

1. A. Flammer, "Self-Efficacy," 5. Also see A. Bandura, "Self-Efficacy."

2. Bandura, "Self-Efficacy."

3. See S. A. Wiedenfeld et al., "Impact of Perceived Self-Efficacy in Coping with Stressors on Components of the Immune System."

4. See B. Knauper, "Symptom Awareness and Interpretation."

5. D. Shapiro, "Psychosocial Aspects of Hypertension."

6. Stanley Schachter and Jerome Singer, "Cognitive, Social, and Physiological Determinants of Emotional State."

7. David Mechanic, *Students under Stress*. See also David Mechanic, "Social Psychological Factors Affecting the Presentation of Bodily Complaints."

8. Mark Zborowski, *People in Pain*; idem, "Cultural Components in Response to Pain."

9. David P. Phillips, et al., "The Hound of the Baskervilles Effect."

10. Theodora Lau, *The Handbook of Chinese Horoscopes.*

11. Phillips et al., "The Hound of the Baskervilles Effect."

12. See Shelley Taylor and Jennifer Crocker, "Schematic Bases of Social Information Processing."

13. Ibid. See also Knauper, "Symptom Awareness," 15357–72.

14. Ibid, 15357; Howard Leventhal and M. Diefenbach, "The Active Side of Illness Cognition."

15. Knauper, "Symptom Awareness," 153–60.

16. Henry Beecher, "Pain in Men Wounded in Battle."

17. See Harold Flor, "Health Psychology of Pain."

18. This distinction is analogous to the distinction between disease and illness.

19. Jennifer Whitson and Adam Galinsky, "Lacking Control Increases Illusory Pattern Perception."

20. Suzanne Kaufman, *Consuming Visions,* 133–34.

21. Ibid.

22. James Pennebaker, *The Psychology of Physical Symptoms.*

23. James Pennebaker and Jean M. Lightner, "Competition of Internal and External Information in an Exercise Setting."

24. Ibid., 3, 21.

25. Ibid., 25–26. A second series of experiments, for example, confirmed the same basic hypothesis but approached it in a different way. Physical exertion was held constant (all participants were asked to run at the same pace on a standard treadmill) while researchers attempted to vary the runner's focus of attention. One group of randomly selected runners was provided with direct feedback that allowed them to listen to themselves breathing as they ran; a second group was played an audiotape of distracting street sounds, such as passing traffic and snippets of conversations between passersby. The results confirmed that the level of symptom reporting was significantly higher for those who listened to themselves breathing than for those who listened to street sounds.

26. James Pennebaker, *Opening Up.*

27. Ibid., 15–17.

28. Ibid., 17.

29. Ibid., 19–20.

30. Ibid., 22–24.

31. Ibid., 23–24.

32. Ibid., 35–37.

33. Ibid., 40.

34. Don C. Fowles, "The Arousal Model."
35. Pennebaker, *Opening Up*, 56.
36. Ibid., 24.
37. Ibid., 113, 175–76.
38. Ibid., 103.
39. I am indebted to Neil Smelser for alerting me to the remarkable similarities between Pennebaker's research, the practices associated with medieval pilgrimage, and modern psychoanalytic theories about hysteria.
40. Sigmund Freud and Josef Breuer, *Studies on Hysteria*, 6.

CODA

1. *Marian Library Newsletter,* 1999.
2. Quoted in Ronald Finucane, *Miracles and Pilgrims*, 40.
3. Anne Harrington, *The Cure Within.*
4. Ibid., 18.
5. Paolo Apolito, *The Internet and the Madonna*, 2, 14. For additional material on this topic see Deidre de la Cruz, "The Work of God in the Age of Mechanical Reproduction," which explores the social and cultural bases of people's susceptibility to accepting electronic accounts of apparitions. This paper was presented as part of the conference "The Vision Thing" held in the summers of 2007 and 2008 at the Center for Advanced Study in the Behavioral Sciences at Stanford University and the Collegium Budapest.
6. Ibid., 41, 3.
7. Ibid., 15, 16.
8. Ibid., 50–51.
9. Jerome Taylor and Simon Caldwell, "Catholics Ordered to Keep Quiet over Virgin Visions."
10. Apolito, *The Internet and the Madonna*, 112.
11. Ibid., 113.
12. Ibid., 119.
13. Ibid., 117.
14. Ibid., 155.
15. Ibid., 155–56.
16. Ibid., 169.
17. Ibid., 77.

APPENDIX: ACCOUNTS OF MIRACLES AT MEDIEVAL SHRINES

1. Emma Mason, *St. Wulfstan of Worcester, c. 1008–1095,* 275.

2. Ibid., 276; J. H. F. Piele, trans., *William of Malmesbury's Life of Saint Wulfstan,* 32–33.

3. Piele, *William of Malmesbury's Life of Saint Wulfstan,* 60–61.

4. Mason, *St. Wulfstan,* 279.

5. Piele, *William of Malmesbury's Life of Saint Wulfstan,* 43–55, 62.

6. Ibid., 45–47, 53.

7. See Aelred of Rievaulx, *The Life of St. Edward, King and Confessor.*

8. Ibid., 18, 115, 117.

9. C. H. Lawrence, ed., *The Life of St. Edmund by Matthew Paris,* 165–67.

10. Herbert Thurston, ed., *The Life of Saint Hugh of Lincoln,* 399–409, 467–83, 565.

11. Daphne Stroud, "Miracles of St. Osmund," 111–14.

BIBLIOGRAPHY

Abbott, Edwin A. *St. Thomas of Canterbury.* 2 vols. London: Adam and Charles Black, 1989.

Ader, Robert. "Conditioned Responses." In *Healing and the Mind,* ed. Bill Moyers, 239–48. New York: Broadway Books, 1993.

———. *Psychoneuroimmunology.* New York: Academic Press, 1981.

Ader, Robert, D.L. Felton, and Nicholas Cohen, eds. *Psychoneuroimmunology,* 3rd. ed., vol. 2. San Diego, CA: Academic Press, 2001.

———."Psychoneuroimmunology." In *International Encyclopedia of the Social and Behavioral Sciences,* ed. Neil Smelser and Paul B. Baltes, 18:12422–28. Amsterdam: Elsevier, 2001.

Aelred of Rievaulx. *The Life of St. Edward, King and Confessor.* Trans. Jerome Bertram. Guildford, U.K.: St. Edward's Press, 1990.

Amanzio, M., A. Pollo, G. Maggi, and F. Benedetti. "Response Variability in Placebo Analgesics: A Role for Non-specific Activiation of Endogenous Opioids." *Pain* 90 (2001): 205–15.

Amundsen, Darrel W. *Medicine, Society, and Faith in the Ancient and Medieval Worlds.* Baltimore: Johns Hopkins University Press, 1996.

Angel, Ronald, and Peggy A. Thoits. "The Impact of Culture on the Cognitive Structure of Illness." *Culture, Medicine and Psychiatry* 11 (1987): 465–49.

Apolito, Paolo. *Apparitions of the Madonna at Oliveto Citra.* Translated by William A. Christian Jr. University Park: Pennsylvania State University Press, 1998.

———. *The Internet and the Madonna: Religious Visionary Experience on the Web.* Chicago: University of Chicago Press, 2005.

Artress, Lauren. *Walking the Sacred Path: Rediscovering the Labyrinth as a Spiritual Practice*. New York: Riverhead Books, 2006.

Attwater, Donald, with Catherine Rachel John. *Penguin Dictionary of Saints*. 3rd ed. London: Penguin, 1995.

Ball, Philip. *Universe of Stone: A Biography of Chartres Cathedral*. New York: HarperCollins, 2008.

Bandura, Albert. "Self-Efficacy." In *Encyclopedia of Human Behavior*, ed. V. S. Ramachaudran, 4:71–81. New York: Academic Press, 1994.

———. "Self-Efficacy and Health." In *International Encyclopedia of the Social and Behavioral Sciences*, ed. Neil Smelser and Paul B. Baltes, 20:13815–20. Amsterdam: Elsevier, 2001.

Barber, Malcolm. *The Two Cities: Medieval Europe, 1050–1320*. London: Routledge, 1992.

Barlow, Frank. *Thomas Becket*. Berkeley: University of California Press, 1986.

Barnes, P.M., E. Powell-Griner, K. McFann, and R.L. Nahin. "Complementary and Alternative Medicine Use among Adults, United States, 2002." Advance data from Vital and Health Statistics, May 27, 2004.

Bausell, R. Barker. *Snake Oil Science: The Truth about Complementary and Alternative Medicine*. New York: Oxford University Press, 2007.

Beecher, Henry K. "Pain in Men Wounded in Battle." *Annals of Surgery* 123 (1946): 96–105.

Bellman, B.L. *The Language of Secrecy: Symbols and Metaphors in Poro Ritual*. New Brunswick, NJ: Rutgers University Press, 1984.

Benedetti, F. "The Opposite Effects of the Opiate Antagonist Naloxone and the Cholecystokinin Antagonist Proglumide on Placebo Analgesia." *Pain* 64 (1996): 535–43.

Benedetti, F., and M. Amanzio, et al. "The Specific Effects of Prior Opioid Exposure on Placebo Analgesia and Placebo Respiratory Depression." *Pain* 75 (1998): 313–19.

Benedetti, F., L. Colloca, E. Torre, M. Lanotte, A. Melcarne, M. Pesare, B. Bergamasco, and L. Lopiano. "Placebo-Responsive Parkinson Patients Show Decreased Activity in Single Neurons of Subthalamic Nucleus." *Nature Neuroscience* 7 (2004): 587–88.

Bengtsson, Tommy. "Mortality: The Great Historical Decline." In *International Encyclopedia of the Social and Behavioral Sciences*, ed. Neil Smelser and Paul B. Baltes, 15:10079–085. Amsterdam: Elsevier, 2001.

Berger, Peter, and Thomas Luckman. *The Social Construction of Reality: A Treatise in the Sociology of Knowledge*. Garden City, NY: Anchor Books, 1966.

Berkman, Lisa, and Leonard Syme. "Social Networks, Host Resistance and Mortality: A Nine-Year Follow-Up Study of Alameda County Residents." *American Journal of Epidemiology* 109 (1979): 186–204.

Berkowitz, L. "Psychology of Aggression in Adulthood." In *International Encyclopedia of the Social and Behavioral Sciences*, ed. Neil J. Smelser and Paul B. Baltes, 1:295–99. Amsterdam: Elsevier, 2001.

Biondi, M. "Effects of Stress on Immune Functions: An Overview." In *Psychoneuorimmunology*, 3rd. ed., ed. Robert Ader, D. L. Felton, and Nicholas Cohen, 2:189–226. San Diego, CA: Academic Press, 2001.

Bishop, Greg D. "Emotions and Health." In *International Encyclopedia of the Social and Behavioral Sciences*, ed. Neil J. Smelser and Paul B. Baltes, 7:4454–59. Amsterdam: Elsevier, 2001.

Blackwell, B., S. S. Bloomfield, and C. R. Buncher. "Demonstration to Medical Students of Placebo Responses and Non-drug Factors." *Lancet* 299, no. 763 (1972): 1279–82.

Board of Science and Education, British Medical Association. *Complementary Medicine*. Oxford: Oxford University Press, 1993.

Boissel, J. P., A. M. Philippon, E. Gauthier, J. Schbath, and J. M. Destors. "Time Course of Long-Term Placebo Therapy Effects in Angina Pectoris." *European Heart Journal* 7, no. 12 (1986): 1030–36.

Bonner, G., D. Rollason, and C. Stancliffe, eds. *St. Cuthbert: His Cult and His Community to A.D. 1200*. Woodbridge, U.K.: Boydell Press, 2002.

Bornstein, Daniel, ed. *A People's History of Christianity*, vol. 4, *Medieval Christianity*. Minneapolis, MN: Fortress Press, 2009.

Bower, Bruce. "Placebo Gives Brain Emotional Break." *Science News*, July 2, 2005, 13.

———. "Thinking the Hurt Away: Expectations Hitch Ride on Pain's Brain Pathway." *Science News*, September 10, 2005.

Braithwaite, A., and P. Cooper. "Analgesic Effects of Branding in Treatment of Headaches." *British Medical Journal* 282, no. 6276 (1981): 1576–78.

Brody, Howard, with Daralyn Brody. *The Placebo Response: How You Can Release the Body's Inner Pharmacy for Better Health*. New York: HarperCollins, 2000.

Brown, Peter. *The Cult of Saints: Its Rise and Function in Latin Christianity*. Chicago: University of Chicago Press, 1981.

Bynum, Caroline Walker. "Bodily Miracles and the Resurrection of the Body." In *Belief in History: Innovative Approaches to European and American Religion*, ed. Thomas Kselman, 68–106. Notre Dame, IN: University of Notre Dame Press, 1991.

Campbell, Joseph. *Pathways to Bliss: Mythology and Personal Transformation.* Novato, CA: New World Library, 2004.

Campbell, Joseph, and Bill Moyers. *The Power of Myth.* New York: Doubleday, 1991.

Cantor, Norman. *In the Wake of the Plague: The Black Death and the World It Made.* New York: Free Press, 2001.

Carey, Benedict. "Do You Believe in Magic?" *New York Times,* January 23, 2007.

Carver, Charles S. "Depression, Hopelessness, Optimism and Health." In *International Encyclopedia of the Social and Behavioral Sciences,* ed. Neil Smelser and Paul B. Baltes, 5:3516–22. Amsterdam: Elsevier, 2001.

Cassell, John. "Social Science Theory as a Source of Hypothesis in Epidemiological Research." *American Journal of Public Health* 54 (1964): 1482–88.

Catholic Pages. www.catholic-pages.com. Accessed August 10, 2009.

Cattaneo, A.D., P.E. Lucchilli, and G. Filippuci. "Sedative Effects of Placebo Treatment." *European Journal of Clinical Pharmacology* 3 (1970): 43–45.

Centers for Disease Control. "Death Rates by Age and Age-Adjusted Death Rates for 15 Leading Causes of Death in 2006: United States, 2006." www.disastercenter.com/cdc.

Chatwin, Bruce. *The Songlines.* New York: Penguin Books, 1991.

Chaucer, Geoffrey. *The Canterbury Tales.* Edited by David Wright. London: Fontana Press, 1996.

Christian, William A. *Person and God in a Spanish Valley.* New York: Seminar Press, 1972.

———. *Apparitions in Late Medieval and Renaissance Spain.* Princeton, NJ: Princeton University Press, 1981.

Cipolla, Carlo M. *Before the Industrial Revolution: European Society and Economy, 1000–1700.* New York: W.W. Norton, 1976.

———. *Faith, Reason and the Plague: A Tuscan Story of the Seventeenth Century.* Brighton, U.K.: Harvester Press, 1979.

———. *Miasmas and Disease: Public Health and the Environment in the Preindustrial Age.* New Haven, CT: Yale University Press, 1992.

Cockayne, Emily. *Hubbub: Filth, Noise, and Stench in England.* New Haven, CT: Yale University Press, 2007.

Coffey, Thomas F., Linda Kay Davidson, and Maryjane Dunn, eds. *The Miracles of Saint James: Liber Sancti Jacobi.* New York: Italica Press, 1996.

Cohen, S.D., W.J. Doyle, D. Skoner, B.S. Rabin, and J.M. Gwaltney. "Social Ties and Susceptibility to the Common Cold." *Journal of the American Medical Association* 277 (1997): 1940–44.

Cohen, S. D., A. J. Tyrrell, and A. P. Smith. "Psychosocial Stress and Suscepti- bility to the Common Cold." *New England Journal of Medicine* 325 (1991): 606–12.

Cohn, Samuel. *The Black Death Transformed.* London: Arnold, 2003.

Coleman, Simon, and John Elsner. *Pilgrimage: Past and Present in the World Reli- gions.* Cambridge, MA: Harvard University Press, 1995.

Coster, Will. "Fear and Friction in Urban Communities during the English Civil War." In *Fear in Early Modern Society,* ed. William Naphy and Penny Roberts, 100–177. Manchester: Manchester University Press, 1997.

Coulton, G. G. *Five Centuries of Religion,* vol. 3, *Getting and Spending.* London: Cambridge University Press, 1936.

Cousineau, Phil. *The Art of Pilgrimage: The Seeker's Guide to Making Travel Sacred.* Berkeley, CA: Conari Press, 2000.

Cousins, Norman. *Anatomy of an Illness.* New York: W. W. Norton, 1995.

Cranston, Ruth. *The Miracle of Lourdes.* New York: Doubleday, 1988.

Crum, Alia, and Ellen Langer. "Mind-Set Matters: Exercise and the Placebo Effect." *Psychological Science* 18, no. 2 (February 2007): 165–71.

Darlington, Reginald R., ed. *The Vita Wulfstani of William of Malmesbury.* Lon- don, 1928.

Dawes, J. D., and J. R. Magilton. "The Cemetery of St. Helen-on-the-Walls, Aldwark." *Archaeology of York* 12, no. 1, 1980.

De Craen, A. J., D. E. Moerman, S. H. Heisterkamp, G. N. Tytgat, J. G. Tijssen, and J. Kleijnen. "Placebo Effect in the Treament of Duodenal Ulcer." *British Journal of Clinical Pharmacology* 48, no. 6 (1999): 853–60.

De la Cruz, Deidre. "The Work of God in the Age of Mechanical Reproduc- tion: Miracles, Modernity, and the Non-disappearance of Religion." Paper presented at the 2008 Summer Institute "The Vision Thing," at the Colle- gium Budapest, Budapest, July 2008.

Delbanco, Thomas. "The Healing Roles of Doctor and Patient." In *Heal- ing and the Mind,* ed. Bill Moyers, 7–23. New York: Broadway Books, 1993.

Dickerson, Sally, Tara Gruenewald, and Margaret Kemeny. "When the Social Self Is Threatened: Shame, Physiology, and Health." *Journal of Personality* 72, no. 6 (December 2004): 1191–216.

Duffin, Jacalyn. *Medical Miracles: Doctors, Saints and Healing the Modern World.* New York: Oxford University Press, 2009.

Duffy, Eamon. *The Stripping of the Altars: Traditional Religion in England c.1400– c.1580.* New Haven, CT: Yale University Press, 1992.

Durkheim, Émile. *The Elementary Forms of Religious Life.* Translated and with an introduction by Karen Fields. New York: Free Press, 1995.

Dyer, Christopher. *Standards of Living in the Later Middle Ages: Social Change in England, c. 1200–1520.* Cambridge: Cambridge University Press, 1989.

———. *Making a Living in the Middle Ages: The People of Britain, 850–1520.* New Haven, CT: Yale University Press, 2002.

Eade, John, and Michael Sallnow. *Contesting the Sacred: The Anthropology of Christian Pilgrimage.* Urbana: University of Illinois Press, 1991.

Effros, Bonnie. "Death and Burial." In *A People's History of Christianity,* vol. 4, *Medieval Christianity,* ed. Daniel Bornstein, 53–74. Minneapolis, MN: Fortress Press, 2009.

Eisenberg, David, Roger B. Davis, Susan L. Ettner, Scott Appel, Sonja Wilkey, Maria van Rompay, and Ronald C. Kessler. "Trends in Alternative Medicine in the United States, 1990–97: Results of a Follow-up National Survey." *Journal of the American Medical Association* 280 (1998): 1569–73.

Eisenberg, Leon. "Disease and Illness: Distinctions between Professional and Popular Ideas of Sickness." *Culture, Medicine, and Psychiatry* 1 (1977): 9–23.

Ekirch, A. Roger. *At Day's Close: Night in Times Past.* New York: W. W. Norton, 2005.

Elm, Susanna. "Captive Crowds: Pilgrims and Martyrs." In *Crowds,* ed. Jeffrey Schnapp and Matthew Tiews, 133–48. Stanford, CA: Stanford University Press, 2006.

Engel, George. "The Need for a New Medical Model." *Science* 196 (1977): 129–36.

Erdmann, Jeanne, and Bryan Christie, illustrator. "The Nocebo Effect." *Science News,* February 28, 2009, 30.

———. "Imagination Medicine." *Science News,* December 20, 2009, 26–29.

Ernst, E., and K. L. Resch. "Concept of True and Perceived Placebo Effects." *British Medical Journal* 311 (1995): 551–52.

Ernst, Edward, and Adrian Furnham. *Complementary Medicine: A Research Perspective.* Chichester, U.K.: Wiley and Sons, 1997.

Evans, Dylan. *Placebo: Mind over Matter in Modern Medicine.* New York: Oxford University Press, 2003.

Evans, Gary W. "Crowding and Other Environmental Stressors." In *International Encyclopedia of the Social and Behavioral Sciences,* ed. Neil Smelser and Paul B. Baltes, 5:3018–22. Amsterdam: Elsevier, 2001.

Fagan, Brian. *The Great Warming: Climate Change and the Rise and Fall of Civilization.* New York: Bloomsbury Press, 2008.

Fauconnier, Gilles. "Conceptual Blending." In *International Encyclopedia of the Social and Behavioral Sciences*, ed. Neil Smelser and Paul Baltes, 4:2495–98. Amsterdam: Elsevier, 2001.

Fauconnier, Gilles, and Mark Turner. *The Way We Think: Conceptual Blending and the Mind's Hidden Complexities*. New York: Basic Books, 2002.

Fawzy I., and N. Fawzy, "Psycho-educational Interventions and Health Outcomes." In *Handbook of Human Stress and Health Outcomes*, ed. Ronald Glaser and Janice K. Kielcot-Glaser. San Diego, CA: Academic Press, 1994.

"Febrile Convulsions." WebMD. http://children.webmd.com/tc/fever-seizures-topic-overview/. Accessed August 10, 2009.

Felten, David. "The Brain and the Immune System." In *Healing and the Mind*, ed. Bill Moyers, 213–37. New York, Broadway Books, 1993.

Fichtenau, Heinrich. *Living in the Tenth Century: Mentalities and Social Order.* Chicago: University of Chicago Press, 1991.

Finucane, Ronald C. *Miracles and Pilgrims: Popular Beliefs in Medieval England.* New York: St. Martin's Press, 1995.

Flammer, A. " Self-Efficacy." In *International Encyclopedia of the Social and Behavioral Sciences*, ed. Neil Smelser and Paul B. Baltes, 20:13812–15. Amsterdam: Elsevier, 2001.

Flor, Harold. "Health Psychology of Pain." In *International Encyclopedia of the Social and Behavioral Sciences*, ed. Neil Smelser and Paul B. Baltes, 16:10990–95. Amsterdam: Elsevier, 2001.

Fowles, Don C. "The Arousal Model: Implications of Gray's Two-Factor Theory for Heart Rate, Electrodermal Activity, and Psychopathy." *Psychophysiology* 17 (1980): 87–104.

Frank, Robert Worth, Jr. "Pilgrimage and Sacral Power." in *Journeys toward God: Pilgrimage and Crusade*, ed. Barbara Sargent-Baur, 31–44. Kalamazoo, MI: Medieval Institute Publications, 1992.

Freedberg, David. *The Power of Images: Studies in the History and Theory of Response.* Chicago: University of Chicago Press, 1989.

French, Katherine. "Parish Life." In *A People's History of Christianity*, vol. 4, *Medieval Christianity*, ed. Daniel Bornstein, 329–57. Minneapolis, MN: Fortress Press, 2009.

Freud, Sigmund, and Josef Breuer. *Studies on Hysteria*. New York: Basic Books, 2004.

Fuente-Fernandez, R. de la, T.J. Ruth, et al. "Expectation and Dopamine Release: Mechanisms of the Placebo Effect in Parkinson's Disease." *Science* 293 (2001): 1164–66.

Fuller, John. *The Day of St. Anthony's Fire.* New York: Macmillan, 1968.

Furnham, Adrian. "Alternative and Complementary Healing Practices." In *International Encyclopedia of the Social and Behavioral Sciences*, ed. Neil Smelser and Paul B. Baltes, 1:404–6. Amsterdam: Elsevier, 2001.

Geary, Patrick. *Furta Sacra: Thefts of Relics in the Central Middle Ages.* Princeton, NJ: Princeton University Press, 1978.

———. *Living with the Dead in the Middle Ages.* Ithaca, NY: Cornell University Press, 1994.

Getz, Faye. *Medicine in the English Middle Ages.* Princeton, NJ: Princeton University Press, 1998.

Gimpel, Jean. *The Cathedral Builders.* New York: Evergreen Books, 1984.

Glaser, Ronald, and Janice. K. Kielcot-Glaser, eds. *Handbook of Human Stress and Immunity.* San Diego, CA: Academic Press, 1994.

Goetz, Hans-Werner. *Life in the Middle Ages: From the Seventh to the Thirteenth Century.* Notre Dame, IN: University of Notre Dame Press, 1993.

Goodich, Michael E. *Violence and Miracle in the Fourteenth Century: Private Grief and Public Salvation.* Chicago: University of Chicago Press, 1995.

———. *Miracles and Wonders: The Development of the Concept of Miracle, 1150–1350.* Aldershot, U.K.: Ashgate, 2007.

Gordon, Eleanora C. "Child Health in the Middle Ages As Seen in the Miracles of Five English Saints, A.D. 1150–1220." *Bulletin of the History of Medicine* 60, no. 4 (Winter 1986): 502–22.

Gordon, H. S., and G. E. Rosenthal. "Impact of Marital Status on Outcomes in Hospitalized Patients: Evidence from an Academic Medical Center." *Archives of Internal Medicine* 155 (1995): 2465–71.

Gottfried, Robert. *The Black Death: Natural and Human Disaster in Medieval Europe.* New York: Free Press, 1983.

Gracely, R. H., W. R. Deeter, P. J. Wolksee, et al. "The Effect of Naloxone on Multidimensional Scales of Postsurgical Pain in Nonsedated Patients." *Society for Neuroscience Abstracts* 5 (1979): 609.

Gracely, R. H., R. Dubner, W. R. Deeter, and P. J. Wolskee. "Clinicians' Expectations Influence Placebo Analgesia." *Lancet* 1, no. 1419 (1985): 43.

Guess, Henry A., Linda Engel, Arthur Kleinman, and John Kusek. *The Science of the Placebo: Toward an Interdisciplinary Research Agenda.* London: BMJ Books, 2002.

Gurevich, Aron. *Medieval Popular Culture: Problems of Belief and Perception.* Cambridge: Cambridge University Press, 1988.

Hahn, R. "The Nocebo Phenomenon: Scope and Foundations." In Anne Harrington, ed., *The Placebo Effect: An Interdisciplinary Exploration*, 56–76. Cambridge, MA: Harvard University Press, 1997.

Hale, J. R. "Violence in the Middle Ages: A Background." In *Violence and Civil Disorder in Italian Cities, 1200–1500*, ed. Lauro Martines, 19–37. Berkeley: University of California Press, 1972.

Hallam, H. E., ed. *The Agrarian History of England and Wales, 1042–1350*. Cambridge: Cambridge University Press, 1988.

Hanawalt, Barbara. *The Ties That Bound: Peasant Families in Medieval England*. New York: Oxford University Press, 1986.

Harrington, Anne, ed. *The Placebo Effect: An Interdisciplinary Exploration*. Cambridge, MA: Harvard University Press, 1997.

———. *The Cure Within: A History of Mind-Body Medicine*. New York: W. W. Norton, 2008.

Harris, Paul L. *The Work of the Imagination: Understanding Children's Worlds*. Oxford: Blackwell Publishers, 2000.

Harris, Ruth. *Lourdes: Body and Spirit in the Secular Age*. New York: Penguin Books, 1999.

Harvey, Barbara. *Living and Dying in England, 1100–1540: The Monastic Experience*. New York: Oxford University Press, 1995.

Hashish, I., and W. Harvey. "Anti-inflammatory Effects of Ultrasound Therapy: Evidence for a Major Placebo Effect." *British Journal of Rheumatology* 25 (1986): 77–81.

Hatcher, John. "Mortality in the Fifteenth Century: Some New Evidence." *Economic History Review* 39 (1986): 19–38.

———. "Monastic Mortality: Durham Priory, 1395–1529." *Economic History Review*, 59, no 4 (2006): 667–87.

———. *The Black Death: A Personal History*. Philadelphia: Da Capo Press, 2008.

Henderson, B. N., and Andrew Baum. "Behavioral Medicine." In *International Encyclopedia of the Social and Behavioral Sciences*, ed. Neil Smelser and Paul B. Baltes, 2:1111–18. Amsterdam: Elsevier, 2001.

Herlihy, David. *The Black Death and the Transformation of the West*. Cambridge, MA: Harvard University Press, 1997.

Hillsboro Free Press (Marion, KS), June 15, 2005.

Hobbes, Thomas. *Leviathan; or, The matter, forme & power of a commonwealth, ecclesiasticall and civill*. (1660). Ed A. R. Waller. Cambridge: Cambridge University Press, 1904.

Holt, Richard. "Society and Population, 600–1300." In *The Cambridge Urban History of Britain*, vol. 1. *600–1540*, ed. David Palliser, 79–104. Cambridge: Cambridge University Press, 2000.

Hróbjartsson, A., and P. Gøtzsche. "Is the Placebo Powerless? An Analysis of Clinical Trials Comparing Placebo with No Treatment." *New England Journal of Medicine* 344 (2001): 1594–602.

———. "Is the Placebo Powerless? Update of a Systematic Review of 52 New Randomized Trials Comparing Placebo with No Treatment." *Journal of Internal Medicine* 256 (2004): 91–100.

Iacono, P., et al. "Placebo Effect in Cardiovascular Clinical Pharmacology." *International Journal of Clinical Pharmacology Research* 12 (1992): 53–56.

Jennings, D. "The Confusion between Disease and Illness in Clinical Medicine." *Canadian Medical Association Journal* 1365, no. 8 (October 1986): 865–70.

John of Salisbury. *Policraticus: Of the Frivolities of Courtiers and the Footprints of Philosophers*. Edited and translated by Cary J. Nederman. Cambridge: Cambridge University Press, 1990.

Jordan, William Chester. *The Great Famine*. Princeton, NJ: Princeton University Press, 1996.

———. *Europe in the High Middle Ages*. New York: Penguin, 2001.

Karasek, Robert, and Töres Theorell, eds. *Healthy Work: Stress, Productivity, and the Reconstruction of Working Life*. New York: Basic Books, 1990.

Kaufman, Suzanne K. *Consuming Visions: Mass Culture and the Lourdes Shrine*. Ithaca, NY: Cornell University Press, 2005.

Kelly, John. *The Great Mortality: An Intimate History of the Black Death, the Most Devastating Plague of All Time*. New York: Harper Perennial, 2005.

Kirsch, I., and G. Saperstein. "Listening to Prozac but Hearing Placebo: A Meta-analysis of Antidepressant Medication." *Prevention and Treatment* 1, article 0002a, 1998. http://journals.apa.org/treatment/volume/pree001002a.html.

Kirsch, I., and L.J. Weixel. "Double-Blind versus Deceptive Administration of Placebo." *Behavioral Neuroscience* 102, no. 2 (1988): 319–23.

Kitayama, Evelyn. "Culture and the Expression of Emotion." In *International Encyclopedia of the Social and Behavioral Sciences*, ed. Neil Smelser and Paul B. Baltes, 5:3134–39. Amsterdam: Elsevier, 2001.

Kleinman, Arthur, Veena Das, and Margaret Lock, eds. *Social Suffering*. Berkeley: University of California Press, 1997.

Knauper, B. "Symptom Awareness and Interpretation." In *International Encyclopedia of the Social and Behavioral Sciences*, ed. Neil Smelser and Paul B. Baltes, 23:15357–62. Amsterdam: Elsevier, 2001.

Kopacz, Krzysztof. "Pilgrims Collect Water at Papal Monument." www.news max.com, August 8, 2006.

Kradin, Richard. *The Placebo Response and the Power of Unconscious Healing.* New York: Routledge, 2008.

Kulielka, B.M., and C. Kirschbaum. "Stress and Health Research." In *International Encyclopedia of the Social and Behavioral Sciences*, ed. Neil Smelser and Paul B. Baltes, 22:15170–78. Amsterdam: Elsevier, 2001.

Kurlansky, Mark. *Salt: A World History.* New York: Penguin Books, 2002.

Labisch, Alfons. "History of Medicine." In *International Encyclopedia of the Social and Behavioral Sciences*, ed. Neil Smelser and Paul B. Baltes, 14:9539–45. Amsterdam: Elsevier, 2001.

Langmuir, G.I. "Thomas of Monmouth: Detector of Ritual Murder." *Speculum* 59 (1984): 820–46.

Lau, Theodora. *The Handbook of Chinese Horoscopes.* 6th ed. New York: Collins, 2007.

Lawrence, C.H., ed. and trans. *The Life of St. Edmund by Matthew Paris.* London: Sandpiper Books, 1996.

Lerner, Michael. "Wounded Healers." In *Healing and the Mind*, ed. Bill Moyers, 323–41. New York: Broadway Books, 1993.

Leuchter, A., I.A. Cook, E.A. Witte, M.L. Morgan, and M. Abrams. "Changes in Brain Function of Depressed Patients during Treatment with Placebo." *American Journal of Psychiatry* 159 (2002): 122–29.

Leventhal, Howard, and M. Diefenbach. "The Active Side of Illness Cognition." In *Mental Representation in Health and Illness*, ed. J.A. Skelton and R.T. Croyle. New York: Springer Verlag, 1991.

Levine, J., N.C. Gordon, and H. Fields, "The Mechanism of Placebo Analgesia." *Lancet* 159 (1978): 654–57.

Lindstrom, L. "The Anthropology of Secrets." In *International Encyclopedia of the Social and Behavioral Sciences*, ed. Neil Smelser and Paul B. Baltes, 20:13780–83. Amsterdam: Elsevier, 2001.

Lock, Margaret. "Ambiguities of Aging: Japanese Experience and Perceptions of Menopause." *Culture, Medicine, and Psychiatry* 10 (1986): 23–46.

Lucchilli, P.E., A.D. Cattaneo, and J. Zattoni. "Effects of Capsule Colour and Order of Administration of Hypnotic Treatments." *European Journal of Clinical Pharmacology* 13 no. 2 (1978): 153–55.

Luhrmann, Tanya. "The Magic of Secrecy." *Ethos* 2 (1989): 131–66.

Malden, A.R., ed. *The Canonization of S. Osmund.* Salisbury: Bennett Brothers, 1901.

Manchester, William. *A World Lit Only by Fire*. Boston: Little, Brown, 1992.

Manuck, S. B., J. R. Kaplan, M. R. Adams, and T. B. Clarkson. "Studies of Psychosocial Influences on Coronary Artery Atherogenesis in Cynomolgus Monkeys." *Health Psychology* 7 (1988): 113–24.

Marian Library Newsletter, 1999.

Marmot, Michael G., H. Bosma, H. Hemingway, et al. "Contributions of Job Control and Other Risk Factors to Social Variations in Coronary Heart Disease Incidence." *Lancet* 350 (1997): 235–39.

Marshall, Peter. "Fear, Purgatory and Polemic in Reformation England." In *Fear in Early Modern Society*, ed. William Naphy and Penny Roberts, 150–66. Manchester: Manchester University Press, 1997.

Martines, Laura, ed. *Violence and Civil Disorder in Italian Cities, 1200–1500*. Berkeley: University of California Press, 1972.

Mason, Emma. *St Wulfstan of Worcester, c. 1008–1095*. Oxford: Oxford University Press, 1990.

Mechanic, David. *Students under Stress: A Study of the Social Psychology of Adjustment*. New York: Free Press, 1962.

———. "Social Psychological Factors Affecting the Presentation of Bodily Complaints. *New England Journal of Medicine* 286 (1972): 1132–39.

———. *Medical Sociology*. 2nd ed. New York: Free Press, 1978.

Melczer, William. *The Pilgrim's Guide to Santiago de Compostela: First English Translation with Introduction, Commentaries and Notes*. New York: Italica Press, 1993.

Miller, Edward, and John Hatcher. *Medieval England: Rural Society and Economic Change, 1086–1348*. London: Longman, 1978.

Moerman, Daniel. "Cultural Variations in the Placebo Effect: Ulcers, Anxiety, and Blood Pressure." *Medical Anthropology Quarterly* 14, no. 1 (2000): 1–22.

———. *Meaning, Medicine and the "Placebo Effect."* Cambridge: Cambridge University Press, 2002.

Montgomery, Guy, and Irving Kirsch. "Mechanisms of Placebo Pain Reduction: An Empirical Investigation." *Psychological Science* 7, no. 3 (1996): 174–76.

Moseley, J. Bruce, K. O'Malley, N. Petersen, T. Menke, B. Brody, D. Kuykendall, J. Hollingsworth, C. Ashton, and N. Wray. "A Controlled Trial of Arthroscopic Surgery for Osteoarthritis of the Knee." *New England Journal of Medicine* 347, no. 2 (July 2002): 81–88.

Moyers, Bill, ed. *Healing and the Mind*. New York: Broadway Books, 1993.

Naphy, William, and Penny Roberts. *Fear in Early Modern Society*. Manchester: Manchester University Press, 1997.

National Center for Health Statistics, *QuickStats: Infant Mortality Rates for 10 Leading Causes of Infant Death . . . : United States, 2005.* www.cdc.gov/mmwr/preview/mmwr.html/mm5642a8.

Neergaard, Lauran. "Expecting Pain Relief Triggers Real Thing." *San Jose Mercury News,* February 20, 2004.

Nemeroff, Carol, and Paul Rozin. "The Makings of the Magical Mind: The Nature and Function of Sympathetic Magical Thinking." In *Imagining the Impossible: Magical, Scientific, and Religious Thinking in Children,* ed. Karl S. Rosengren, Carl N. Johnson, and Paul L. Harris, 1–34. Cambridge: Cambridge University Press, 2000.

Nickell, Joe. *Looking for a Miracle: Weeping Icons, Relics, Stigmata, Visions and Healing Cures.* Buffalo, NY: Prometheus Books, 1993.

Nilson, Ben. *Cathedral Shrines of Medieval England.* Woodbridge, U.K.: Boydell Press, 1998.

Nirenberg, David. *Communities of Violence: Persecution of Minorities in the Middle Ages.* Princeton, NJ: Princeton University Press, 1996.

Nisbett, Richard, and Dov Cohen. *Culture of Honor: The Psychology of Violence in the South.* Boulder, CO: Westview, 1996.

Olds, Katrina. "The 'False Chronicles' in Early Modern Spain: Forgery, Tradition, and the Invention of Texts and Relics, 1595–c. 1670." PhD thesis, Princeton University, 2009.

Orth-Gomér, K. "Social Support and Health." In *International Encyclopedia of the Social and Behavioral Sciences,* ed. Neil Smelser and Paul B. Baltes, 21:14452–58. Amsterdam: Elsevier, 2001.

Palliser, David. *The Cambridge Urban History of Britain,* vol. 1, *600–1540.* Cambridge: Cambridge University Press, 2000.

Panofsky, Erwin. *Abbot Suger: On the Abbey Church of St.-Denis and its Art Treasures.* Princeton, NJ: Princeton University Press, 1946.

Pennebaker, James W. *The Psychology of Physical Symptoms.* New York: Springer, 1982.

———. *Opening Up: The Healing Power of Expressing Emotions.* New York: Guilford Press, 1990.

Pennebaker, James W., and J.M. Lightner. "Competition of Internal and External Information in an Exercise Setting." *Journal of Personality and Social Psychology* 39 (1980): 165–74.

Pert, Candace. "The Chemical Communicators." In Bill Moyers, *Healing and the Mind,* 177–93. New York: Broadway Books, 1993.

Peterson, C. "Explanatory Style and Health." In *International Encyclopedia of the Social and Behavioral Sciences*, ed. Neil Smelser and Paul B. Baltes, 8:5162–64. Amsterdam: Elsevier, 2001.

Petrie, Keith J. "Social Support and Recovery from Disease and Medical Procedures." In *International Encyclopedia of the Social and Behavioral Sciences*, ed. Neil Smelser and Paul B. Baltes, 21:14458–61. Amsterdam: Elsevier, 2001.

Phillips, David P., George C. Liu, Kennon Kwok, Jason R. Jarvinen, Wei Zhang, and Ian Abramson. "The Hound of the Baskervilles Effect: Natural Experiment on the Influence of Psychological Stress on Timing of Death." *British Medical Journal* 323, no. 7327 (December 2001): 1443–49.

Piele, J. H. F., trans. *William of Malmesbury's Life of Saint Wulfstan*. Oxford: Basil Blackwell, 1934.

Pitt-Rivers, J. "Honor and Social Status." In *Honour and Shame: The Values of Mediterranean Society*, ed. J. G. Peristiary, 8–77. London: Weidenfeld and Nicholson, 1965.

Plassman, Hilke, John O'Doherty, Baba Shiv, and Antonio Rangel. "Marketing Actions Can Modulate Neural Representations of Experienced Pleasantness." *Proceedings of the National Academy of Sciences* 105, no. 3 (January 2008): 1050–54.

Platt, Colin. *King Death: The Black Death and Its Aftermath in Late-Medieval England*. Toronto: University of Toronto Press, 1966.

Pollo, Antonella, Martina Amanzio, Anna Arslanian, Caterina Casadio, Giuliano Maggi, and Fabrizio Benedetti. "Response Expectancies in Placebo Analgesia and Their Clinical Relevance." *Pain* 93 (2001): 77–84.

Porter, Roy. *London: A Social History*. Cambridge, MA: Harvard University Press, 2001.

Price, D. D. et al. "An Analysis of Factors That Contribute to the Magnitude of Placebo Analgesia in an Experimental Paradigm." *Pain* 83 (1999): 147–56.

Radding, Charles, and William Clark. *Medieval Architecture, Medieval Learning: Builders and Masters in the Age of Romanesque and Gothic*. New Haven, CT: Yale University Press, 1992.

Rawcliffe, Carole. *Medicine and Society in Later Medieval England*. Stroud, U.K.: Sutton Publishing, 1997.

———. *Leprosy in Medieval England*. Woodbridge, U.K.: Boydell Press, 2006.

"Retinoids." WebMD. www.webmd.com/vitamins-lifestyle-guide/supplement-guide/vitamin-a/. Accessed August 10, 2009.

Riley, James. *Rising Life Expectancy: A Global History.* Cambridge: Cambridge University Press, 2001.

Roberts, Geoffrey, ed. *The History and Narrative Reader.* New York: Routledge, 2001.

Roberts, Penny. "Agencies Human and Divine." In *Fear in Early Modern Society,* ed. William Naphy and Penny Roberts, 9–27. Manchester: Manchester University Press, 1997.

Robinson, James Cragie, ed. *Materials for the History of Thomas Becket, Archbishop of Canterbury.* 6 vols. London: Longman and Company, 1875.

Rosengren, A., K. Orth-Gomér, H. Wedel, and L. Wilhelmser. "Stressful Life Events, Social Support, and Mortality in Men Born in 1933." *British Medical Journal* 307 (1993): 1102–5.

Rosengren, Karl S., Carl N. Johnson, and Paul L. Harris, eds. *Imagining the Impossible: Magical, Scientific, and Religious Thinking in Children.* Cambridge: Cambridge University Press, 2000.

Rudolph, Conrad. *Pilgrimage to the End of the World: The Road to Santiago de Compostela.* Chicago: University of Chicago Press, 2004.

Russell, Josiah Cox. *British Medieval Population.* Albuquerque: University of New Mexico Press, 1948.

———. "Populations in Europe, 500–1500." In *Fontana Economic History of Europe,* vol. 1, *The Middle Ages,* ed. Carlo Cipolla, 25–71. Glasgow: Collins/Fontana, 1972.

Sallis, R.E., and L.W. Buckalew. "Relation of Capsule Color and Perceived Potency." *Perceptual and Motor Skills* 58, no. 3 (1984): 897–98.

Sargent-Baur, Barbara, ed. *Journeys toward God: Pilgrimage and Crusade.* Kalamazoo, MI: Medieval Institute Publications, 1992.

Sauro, Menchetti. "Endogenous Opiates and the Placebo Effect: A Meta-analysis Review." *Journal of Psychosomatic Research* 58 (2005): 115–20.

Schachter, Stanley, and Jerome Singer. "Cognitive, Social, and Physiological Determinants of Emotional State." *Psychological Review* 69 (1962): 379–99.

Schapira, K., H.A. McClelland, N.R. Griffiths, and D.J. Newell. "Study on the Effects of Tablet Colour on the Treatment of Anxiety States." *British Medical Journal* 2 (1970): 446–49.

Schnapp, Jeffrey, and Matthew Tiews, eds. *Crowds.* Stanford, CA: Stanford University Press, 2006.

Schofield, Phillipp R. *Peasant and Community in Medieval England, 1200–1500.* Basingstoke, U.K.: Palgrave MacMillan, 2007.

Schutte, Anne Jacobson. *Aspiring Saints: Pretense of Holiness, Inquisition, and Gender in the Republic of Venice, 1618–1750*. Baltimore, MD: Johns Hopkins University Press, 2001.

Scott, Robert A. *The Gothic Enterprise: A Guide to Understanding the Medieval Cathedral*. Berkeley: University of California Press, 2003.

Scott, Robert A., Linda H. Aiken, David Mechanic, and Julius Moravcsik. "Organizational Aspects of Caring." *Millbank Quarterly* 73, no. 1 (1995): 77–96.

Scott, Susan, and Christopher Duncan. *Return of The Black Death: The World's Greatest Serial Killer*. Chichester, U.K.: Wiley and Sons, 2004.

Shahar, Shulamith. *Childhood in the Middle Ages*. London: Routledge, 1990.

Shampan'er, Kristina, and Dan Ariely. "Zero as a Special Price: The True Value of Free Products." *Marketing Science* 26, no. 6 (2007): 742–57.

Shapiro, Arthur, and Elaine Shapiro. *The Powerful Placebo: From Ancient Priest to Modern Physician*. Baltimore, MD: Johns Hopkins University Press, 1997.

Shapiro, D. "Psychosocial Aspects of Hypertension." In *International Encyclopedia of the Social and Behavioral Sciences*, ed. Neil Smelser and Paul B. Baltes, 10:7098–101. Amsterdam: Elsevier, 2001.

Simmel, George. "The Secret and the Secret Society." In *The Sociology of George Simmel*, ed. K. Wolff. Glencoe, IL: Free Press, 1950.

Siraisi, Nancy G. *Medieval and Early Renaissance Medicine: An Introduction to Knowledge and Practice*. Chicago: University of Chicago Press, 1997.

Smelser, Neil. *The Odyssey Experience*. Berkeley: University of California Press, 2009.

Smelser, Neil, and Paul B. Baltes, eds. *International Encyclopedia of the Social and Behavioral Sciences*. 26 vols. Amsterdam: Elsevier, 2001.

Smith, T. W. "Health Psychology." In *International Encyclopedia of the Social and Behavioral Sciences*, ed. Neil Smelser and Paul B. Baltes, 10:6602–8. Amsterdam: Elsevier, 2001.

Steptoe, Andrew. "Infectious Diseases: Psychosocial Aspects." In *International Encyclopedia of the Social and Behavioral Sciences*, ed. Neil Smelser and Paul B. Baltes, 11:7422–27. Amsterdam: Elsevier, 2001.

Sternberg, Esther. *Healing Spaces: The Science of Place and Well-Being*. Cambridge, MA: Belknap Press of Harvard University Press, 2009.

Stokols, Daniel. "Ecology and Health." In *International Encyclopedia of the Social and Behavioral Sciences*, ed. Neil Smelser and Paul B. Baltes, 6:4030–35. Amsterdam: Elsevier, 2001.

Stroud, Daphne. "Miracles of St. Osmund." *Hatcher Review* 3, no. 23 (Spring 1987): 107–15.

Sumption, Jonathan. *The Age of Pilgrimage: The Medieval Journey to God.* Mahwah, NJ: HiddenSpring, 1975.

Swanson, R.N. *Religion and Devotion, c. 1215-c. 1515.* Cambridge: Cambridge University Press, 1995.

Syme, S.L. "Social Epidemiology." In *International Encyclopedia of the Social and Behavioral Sciences,* ed. Neil Smelser and Paul B. Baltes, 7:4701–6. Amsterdam: Elsevier, 2001.

Talbot, Margaret. "The Placebo Prescription." *New York Times Magazine,* January 9, 2000.

Taylor, Jerome, and Simon Caldwell. "Catholics Ordered to Keep Quiet over Virgin Visions." *Independent,* January 13, 2009.

Taylor, Margery. *Imaginary Companions and the Children Who Create Them.* New York: Oxford University Press, 2001.

Taylor, Shelley, and Jennifer Crocker. "Schematic Bases of Social Information Processing." In *Social Cognition: Ontario Symposium on Personality and Social Psychology,* ed. E. T. Higgins et al. Hillsdale, NJ: Erlbaum, 1978.

Thacker, Alan. "Lindisfarne and the Origins of the Cult of St. Cuthbert." In *St. Cuthbert: His Cult and His Community to A.D. 1200,* ed. G. Bonner, D. Rollason, and C. Stancliffe, 103–22. Woodbridge, U.K.: Boydell Press, 2002.

Thomas, Keith. *Religion and the Decline of Magic.* New York: Charles Scribner's Sons, 1971.

Thomas, Lewis. "On Warts." In *The Medusa and the Snail: More Notes of a Biology Watcher,* 76–81. New York: Viking Press, 1979.

Thurston, Herbert, trans. and ed. *The Life of Saint Hugh of Lincoln.* London: Burns and Oates, 1898.

Tinniswood, Adrian. *By Permission of Heaven: The True Story of the Great Fire of London.* New York: Riverhead Books, 2004.

Torrance, Robert. *The Spiritual Quest: Transcendence in Myth, Religion, and Science.* Berkeley: University of California Press, 1994.

Torrance, W.J. *The Life of St. Osmund.* London: Skeffington and Son, Ltd., 1920.

Tuchman, Barbara. *A Distant Mirror: The Calamitous Fourteenth Century.* New York: Ballantine Books, 1978.

Tudor, Victoria. "The Cult of St. Cuthbert in the 12th Century: The Evidence of Reginald of Durham." In *St. Cuthbert: His Cult and His Community to A.D. 1200,* ed. G. Bonner, D. Rollason, and C. Stancliffe, 447–68. Woodbridge, U.K.: Boydell Press, 2002.

Turner, Victor, and Edith Turner. *Image and Pilgrimage in Christian Culture.* New York: Columbia University Press, 1978.

Tweedie, R.L. "Meta-analysis: Overview." In *International Encyclopedia of the Social and Behavioral Sciences*, ed. Neil Smelser and Paul B. Baltes, 14:9717–24. Amsterdam: Elsevier, 2001.

Van Dam, Raymond. *Saints and Their Miracles in Late Antique Gaul*. Princeton, NJ: Princeton University Press, 1978.

Vauchez, André. *Sainthood in the Later Middle Ages*. Trans. Jean Birrel. Cambridge: Cambridge University Press, 1997.

Vickers, A.J. "Can Acupuncture Have Specific Effects on Health? A Systematic Review of Acupuncture Antiemesis Trials." *Journal of the Royal Society of Medicine* 89, no. 6 (1996): 303–11.

Vincent, C., and A. Furnham. *Complementary Medicine: A Research Perspective*. Chichester, U.K.: Wiley, 1997.

Wager, T.D., J.K. Rilling, E.E. Smith, et al. "Placebo-Induced Changes in fMRI in the Anticipation and Experience of Pain." *Science* 303 (2004): 1162.

Wakin, Daniel. "Cardinals Lobby for Swift Sainthood for John Paul II." *New York Times*, April 12, 2005.

Webb, Diana. *Medieval European Pilgrimage, c. 700–c. 1500*. Basingstoke, U.K.: Palgrave, 2002.

Weber, Max. *The Sociology of Religion*. Translated by Talcott Parsons. Boston: Beacon Press, 1993.

Welin, L., K. Svardsudd, S. Ander-Perciva, et al. "Prospective Study of Social Influences on Mortality: The Study of Men Born in 1913 and 1923." *Lancet* 325 (1985): 915–18.

White, Hayden. "The Historical Text as Literary Artifact." In *The History and Narrative Reader*, ed. Geoffrey Roberts, 221–36. New York: Routledge, 2001.

White, L., B. Tursky, and G.E. Schwartz. *Placebo: Theory, Research, and Mechanisms*. New York: Guilford Press, 1985.

Whitson, Jennifer, and Adam Galinsky. "Lacking Control Increases Illusory Pattern Perception." *Science* 322 (October 2008): 115–17.

Wiech, Katja, Miguel Farias, Guy Kahane, Nicholas Shackel, Wiebke Tiede, and Irene Tracey. "An fMRI Measuring Analgesia Enhanced by Religion as a Belief System." *Pain* 139, no. 2 (2008): 467–76.

Wiedenfeld, S.A., A. Bandura, A. O'Leary, S. Brown, and K. Raska. "Impact of Perceived Self-Efficacy in Coping with Stressors on Components of the Immune System." *Journal of Personality and Social Psychology* 59 (1990): 1082–94.

Wolfe, Michael, ed. *One Thousand Roads to Mecca: Ten Centuries of Travelers Writing about the Muslim Pilgrimage*. New York: Grove Press, 1997.

Wrigley, E. A., and R. S. Schofield. *The Population History of England, 1541–1871.* Cambridge: Cambridge University Press, 2005.

Yarrow, Simon. *Saints and Their Communities: Miracle Stories in Twelfth-Century England.* Oxford: Oxford University Press, 2006.

Zborowski, Mark. "Cultural Components in Responses to Pain." *Journal of Social Issues* 4 (1952): 16–30.

———. *People in Pain.* San Francisco: Jossey-Bass, 1969.

Zeigler, Philip. *The Black Death.* Stroud, U.K.: Sutton, 1969.

Zimdars-Swartz, Sandra L. *Encountering Mary: From La Salette to Medjugorje.* Princeton, NJ: Princeton University Press, 1991.

Zubieta, Jon-Kar, et al. "Placebo Effects Mediated by Endogenous Opioid Activity on M-Opioid Receptors." *Journal of Neuroscience* 24 (August 2005): 7754–62.

INDEX

Page numbers in italics indicate illustrations.

Compositor: BookComp Inc.
Text: 10/15 Janson
Display: Janson
Indexer: J. Naomi Linzer Indexing Services
Cartographer: Bill Nelson
Printer/Binder: Maple-Vail Book Manufacturing Group